Neuroscience Research Progress

nova
Medicine & Health
New York

Neuroscience Research Progress

The Dentate Gyrus: Structure, Functions and Health Implications
Feng-Ru Tang, PhD, MD (Editor)
2021. ISBN: 978-1-68507-212-4 (Hardcover)
2021. ISBN: 978-1-68507-240-7 (eBook)

Systemic, Cellular and Molecular Mechanisms of Physiological Functions and Their Disorders (Proceedings of I. Beritashvili Center for Experimental Biomedicine – 2021)
Nargiz Nachkebia, PhD
Nodar P. Mitagvaria, PhD, Dr. of Sci.
(Editors)
2021. ISBN: 978-1-68507-113-4 (Hardcover)
2021. ISBN: 978-1-68507-135-6 (eBook)

Neuromanagement: Neuroscience for Organizations
Michela Balconi (Editor)
2021. ISBN: 978-1-53619-562-0 (Hardcover)
2021. ISBN: 978-1-53619-650-4 (eBook)

Understanding Children with Attention Deficit Hyperactivity Disorder (ADHD)
Janna Glozman (Editor)
2020. ISBN: 978-1-53618-224-8 (Hardcover)
2020. ISBN: 978-1-53618-231-6 (eBook)

Unlocking Erik: A Freedom Journey to Restore the Speech of Those with Locked-In Syndrome
Philip R. Kennedy, MD, PhD (Editor)
2020. ISBN: 978-1-53617-455-7 (Softcover)
2020. ISBN: 978-1-53617-487-8 (eBook)

More information about this series can be found at https://novapublishers.com/product-category/series/neuroscience-research-progress/

Prachi Srivastava, PhD
Neha Srivastava, PhD
and Prekshi Garg
Editors

New Perspectives in Neuroscience

nova
Medicine & Health
New York

DOI: https://doi.org/10.52305/MEHM5624

Library of Congress Cataloging-in-Publication Data

ISBN: 978-1-68507-754-9

Published by Nova Science Publishers, Inc. † New York

Contents

Preface

Neuroscience is a complex and important part of human physiology as it governs all the important actions of life. The complexity of the brain makes it challenging, yet interesting, to decode its information through different mechanistic approaches. Scientists and researchers always remain curious in finding out new avenues related to neuroscience. The main purpose of this book is to bring all relevant and current advancements occurring in the field of neurobiology and neurosciences under a single window that covers wider horizons of the subject. The book contains topics related to subjects like neuro-epigenetics, neuro-informatics, neurotoxicity, neurolaw, neuro-dental issues, neuro-transcriptomics, neuro-nanotechnology and more that focus on the current trends of neurosciences. Nearly all current aspects of neurosciences are covered in this book, which makes it a unique and comprehensive compilation. Chapter One defines different aspects of neuroinformatics; Chapter Two signifies the ongoing trends related to bioinformatics in the field of neurosciences; Chapter Three speaks about neurotoxicity; Chapter Four is a landmark in defining the computational approaches that can be used for the identification of novel biomarkers for neurological disorders; Chapter Five describes in detail about the role of miRNA in neurobiology; Chapter Six illustrates in detail the application of epigenetics in neurological disorders; Chapter Seven covers the details of the therapies that are used for the treatment of neurodegenerative diseases; Chapter Eight is confined to Alzheimer's disease and its mitophagy, autophagy and angiogenesis; Chapter Nine discusses the role of neuro-nanotechnology in neurosurgery; Chapter Ten depicts the dental care that should be given to patients who are suffering from neurological diseases; Chapter Eleven signifies the current trends that are prevalent in the field of oral neurosciences; and Chapter Twelve is focused on the legal perspectives of neuroscience, that is, neurolaw.

Therefore, the coverage of subject in relation to the current trends is quite wide and the book covers a holistic approach in linearity with its title and content.

Chapter 1

Bioinformatics Application and Progress in Therapeutic Interventions of Neurological Disorders

Vishal M. Balaramnavar[1], Deepti Mathpal[1], Prachi Srivastava[2] and Khurshid Ahmad[3,*]

[1]School of Pharmacy and Research Centre, Sanskriti University, Mathura, U.P., India
[2]AMITY Institute of Biotechnology, AMITY University Uttar Pradesh, Lucknow, U.P., India
[3]Department of Medical Biotechnology, Yeungnam University, Gyeongsan, Republic of Korea

Abstract

The brain is concerned with the entire development and functioning of the complex system, as well as the development of its type. Bioinformatics is involved in the development and application of novel informatics in the biological sciences.

This chapter will benefit the clinical domain by offering current knowledge in the field of clinical neurosciences, such as database construction and methods for analyzing crucial data from the massive amount of clinical research and treatment data available to the scientific community.

---

* Corresponding Author's Email: ahmadk@ynu.ac.kr.

In: New Perspectives in Neuroscience
Editors: Prachi Srivastava, Neha Srivastava and Prekshi Garg
ISBN: 978-1-68507-754-9

It also offers an overview of the subjects of neuroscience, computational neuroscience, and neuroinformatics, as well as reasonable approaches or procedures in software tools and resources.

Keywords: neurosciences, neuroinformatics, neurological disorders, neuroscience databases

Introduction

The brain is certainly a vibrant, adaptive organ. Throughout childhood and adolescence, our brain grows in response to complex interactions of genetic and environmental influences, and it has a capability for functional and structural rearrangement even in maturity. Neuroscience research is now providing a plethora of comprehensive information about the many characteristics of cells and circuits that underpin mammalian brain processes [1]. Informatics tools will be necessary to reach the scientific community's failure to address the humongous amounts of new data collected in neuroscience, where the physiological outcome, biochemical status, physiological parameters, genetic data, subcellular, and cellular (along with all advanced studies such as epigenetics, metabolomics, and transcriptomics) must be linked in a comprehensible manner [2].

The human brain is concerned with the overall development and functions of the complex system even for its kind. The coding and modeling for analysis of neurons approximately 86.1 ± 8.1 billion neurons and equally glial cells along with 100 trillion connections are needed [3]. The field is very recent advance to the area and it describes a few innovative applications in detecting the brain network, organization, predicting disorder diagnosis, and simulation analysis using the computer. The system is comprised of a brain-system and system-brain interface along with a brain-to-brain interface. It also provides an integrated overview of fields in an opposite approach for general literature and a nontechnical way for entering this field.

Brain consists of 13% of global disease set for neurological disorders which are far more than cardiovascular disease amounting to 5% of global disease and 10% of different cancers constituted the global disease sets [4]. In the present scenario, neuroscience is multidisciplinary science comprised of bioinformaticians, doctors, molecular biologists, psychologists, computer scientists, clinicians, engineers, theoretical and experimental physicists, mathematicians, and philosophers among others. Therefore, it is a diverse mix of researchers who give a glance at the rich radiance of this field. The nervous systems manipulate and process the information very fast. The mathematical theory with different positions and relations is desirable for computing the outputs from the nervous system. The computational models were needed for hypothetical modeling [5]. The neuronal signal is a different kind of computational signal and its not been calculated as digital or analog [6]. The nervous system can be decomposed number of subsystems like the cortex and brainstem. The subsystems can be further divided into smaller systems leading to the formation of computational neurosciences. The approach leads to the generation of highly complex data in huge capacity. Storage, information extraction, data analysis, and quick dispersal. The computer-based data management and presentation data are required steps in the analysis of neurological data.

These areas finally resulted in a new integrated branch of neuro-informatics [7]. Neuroinformatics study involved the development of processes for data storage, infrastructure, and sophisticated tools for the development of the superior tools for data extraction and dispersion and methods for analyzing such data which may assist major advancements in understanding the structural and functional aspects of the human brain [8].

The computational part is followed by analyzing applications and challenges of neuroinformatics research along with a few data sources, tools and software, simulation platforms, existing languages, a few innovative applications.

Computational Neurosciences and Neuroinformatics

The study of the brain to discover the principles of the brain and mechanisms to control the nervous system's development, processing the collected information and mental capacities.

Computational neuroscience is dependent on biology aided with computational tools and software, physics, mathematics, and is the answer to a huge amount of data in form of clinical records, literature to form neuroinformatics. Thus, it is an interface between computer science and neuronal science. It is the study of brain connections/networks to discover the brain network and its activities according to explicit information and structural as well as functional properties of the brain using computational techniques [9].

The main advantage of computational neuroscience is to explore the process of illustration and exploitation of information in the brain using electrical and chemical signals.

The normal activities of the brain include hearing, seeing, remembering, and controlling by simulating neuronal systems and large brain networks with the advancement of computational power. In an era of rapidly growing cross-disciplinary knowledge, neuroinformatics is becoming increasingly important to neuroscience researchers and clinicians for pursuing scientific inquiry and practicing medicine [10].

Neuroscience Databases and Tools

There are several neuroscience databases and resources available to help understand neuroscience and biomedicine. Neuroinformatics can be thought of as an expanded and elaborated application of comparable methods proven crucial for the development of bioinformatics but applied to a bigger, heterogeneous set of data at multiple levels of function. The neuroscience community has benefited from several attempts to develop web-based databases. Some enable morphometric and time-series data input, as well as linkages to compartmental modeling and scientific visualization [11, 12].

The Allen Institute for Brain Science (https://portal.brain-map.org/) takes a novel method to generate data, tools, and information for scholars investigating the mammalian brain's biological complexities. This portal gives researchers throughout the world access to high-quality data and web-based tools. The web portal contains specifically, *New Data and Tools* to explore mouse patch-seq data from approximately 3600 mouse cortical neurons, and brain observatory (Visual Behavior - 2P). *Allen Brain Atlases and Data* includes a cell types database based on multimodal characterization of single cells, as well as a database of neuronal cell types.

BrainMaps.org (http://brainmaps.org/) is an immersive, next-generation brain atlas built on over 140 million megapixels of sub-micron resolution, compiled, scanned images of serial sections of primate and non-primate brains and integrated with a high-speed database for querying and retrieving data about brain structure and function over the internet.

Mouse Brain Proteome (http://www.mousebrainproteome.com/) provides an in-depth study of the mouse brain and its key brain areas and cell types using high-resolution mass spectrometry-based proteomics.

The NeuroImaging Tools & Resources Collaboratory (https://www.nitrc.org/) is an internet resource that provides detailed information on a wide range of neuroinformatics tools and data. NITRC has aided neuroscience research in making discoveries by utilizing software and data generated from previously abandoned or ignored research. It also allows for free data access as well as pay-per-use cloud-based accessibility to infinite computing capacity, allowing for global scientific collaboration with little setup and cost. The Resources Registry (NITRC-R), Image Repository (NITRC-IR), and Computational Environment (NITRC-CE) are all components of NITRC (NITRC-CE).

Several additional neural databases are open to the public and contain up-to-date information as well as pertinent references. For example, SenseLab (https://senselab.med.yale.edu/) is a collection of 10 databases that enable experimental and theoretical study on the membrane characteristics that mediate information processing in nerve cells, with the olfactory pathway serving as a model system. Neuronal, olfactory, and diseases are the three categories. All of the databases have the same database structure, allowing for seamless navigation between them. The neural databases include tools for searching for combinations of characteristics across different neuron types. The olfactory databases are primarily concerned with olfactory receptors and odor mapping.

Another webpage to browse and understand brain experimental data is "CRCNS - Collaborative Research in Computational Neuroscience" (https://crcns.org/), which serves as a marketplace and conversation platform for integrating neuroscience tools and data [13]. The Neuroscience Information Framework (https://neuinfo.org//) is a dynamic database of neuroscience data, resources, and tools available on the Internet. It is a meta-database of over 100 databases including neuroscience-relevant data from humans, mice, rats, and worms.

Computer Aided Drug Design (CADD)

CADD is a wide term that refers to a variety of theoretical and computational techniques used in current drug development. Computational chemistry, molecular modeling, molecular design, and rational drug design are all part of it. CADD encompasses a wide range of computational methods such as direct and indirect virtual screening, library design, lead optimization, and de novo design, among others [14]. Chemical biology and computational drug design techniques are used in drug development to efficiently identify and optimize lead molecules. CADD's success has led to its recognition as an essential technology in the field of research and pharmaceuticals [15].

Application of CADD in Treatment of Neurological Disorders

Neurodegenerative disorders (NDs) are a group of diseases that are untreatable, disturbing, and are defined by the progressive structural and functional loss of neurons. NDs are generally arise with age or aging of cells and socioeconomic burdens. Alzheimer's disease (AD), Parkinson's disease (PD), Huntington's disease (HD), and amyotrophic lateral sclerosis (ALS) are only a few of the major neurodegenerative conditions [16]. These disorders are related to dementia which is a collection of symptoms associated with impairment of cognitive specifically related to memory function and interfere with normal functioning [17]. There are numerous examples of CADD being used successfully for the management of NDs [16, 18-20].

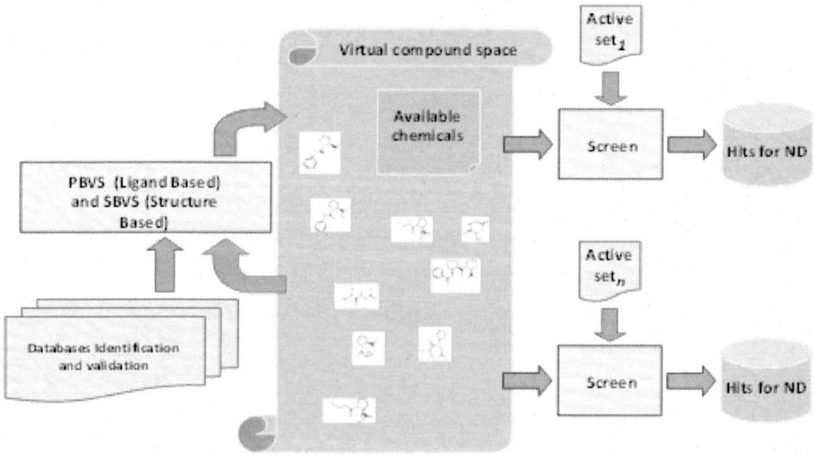

Figure 1. Workflow for the screening of chemical compounds for the management of neurological disorders (NDs) [21, 22].

The computational models simplify the complexity of the disease and also offered a bridge across species. The use of artificial intelligence (AI) models, data-driven computational, statistical models may help in mapping the relationships crosswise symptoms and markers but also act as a clinical verdict to support systems by providing more objective and standardized information regarding status or progression. The development of a computational or statistical model would require the availability of a huge database from available resources. The databases like Neuroimaging Initiative (ADNI), the National Alzheimer's Coordinating Center (NACC), and the Dementias Platform UK (DPUK). These open datasets now enable researchers, particularly, those with a computational or theoretical incline, to perform large-scale quantitative analyses to enable bigger research impact.

This approach involving the quantitative and computational methods can be applied to address some of the previously mentioned issues. The part is classified under the Computational Neurology section. The first section will discuss mechanistic modeling through Computational Neuroscience, and the second section will be on data-driven approaches. Figure 1 summarizes these computational approaches.

Alzheimer's Disease (AD)

Amyloid-beta (Aβ) is a vital therapeutic target in AD. An in-silico technique was used to examine a series of peptides against the fibrillar form of Aβ, and two active compounds were found [23].

These peptides were later discovered to prevent the neurotoxic effects of Aβ on neuroblastoma cells. BACE-1 is an enzyme that has been shown to be required for the generation of Aβ [24]. Inhibiting BACE suppresses the formation of Aβ and hence prevents NDs like AD [25], implying that BACE-1 is an avital therapeutic target for NDs.

The structural behavior of BACE-1 has been studied using a variety of computational methods, as well as the design of inhibitors [26]. ROCK-I and NOX2 are two of the most appealing prospective therapeutic targets for different NDs [27, 28], and their inhibition is used to treat neurological disorders such as autism spectrum disease, AD, and fragile X syndrome. CADD has been used successfully to develop dual inhibitors for these enzymes by combining pharmacophores and utilizing a molecular docking technique to discover chemical entities [29]. The inhibitory potential of selected chemical entities against ROCK-I and NOX2 was established in vitro. Acetylcholinesterase (AChE) inhibitors have been proposed as possible treatments for AD.

The binding of chemicals identified in *Salvia miltiorrhiza* extracts, such as miltirone and salvianolic acid A, to AChE[30], as well as the binding of cinerin C (derived from *Prosopis cineraria* pods), to AChEhave been described using molecular docking [31].

Parkinson's Disease (PD)

PD is the second most prevalent ND, characterized by tremors, muscle rigidity, and postural imbalance [32, 33]. Catecholsare metabolized by Catechol-O-Methyltransferase (COMT) through methylation.

COMT is considered a therapeutic target for the treatment of PD since dopamine is one of the catechols that is decreased in the CNS throughout the disease.

Structure-based drug design studies identified nitrocatechol-type inhibitors (tolcapone and entacapone), bisubstrate inhibitors (thiopyridine, purine, N-methyladenine, and 6-methylpurine), and other compounds (4-phenyl-7, 8-dihydroxycoumarin) as possible COMT inhibitors [34].

Amyotrophic Lateral Sclerosis (ALS)

ALS is a fatal disease that causes progressive muscular paralysis and wasting. It is caused by the loss of neurons that regulate voluntary muscles, including upper motor neurons in the motor cortex and lower motor neurons in the brainstem and spinal cord [35]. Variations in zinc and copper ion binding to Superoxide dismutase (SOD1) cause misfolded enzymes, which can contribute to aggregation and ALS-related protein instability. With the goal of discovering lead compounds for ALS, 32,791 molecules were virtually screened using the *in silico* technique for inhibitors of the abnormal interaction between mutant SOD1 and tubulin [36]. CADD studies have indicated a variety of inhibitors like linear tripeptides [37], the tubulin-binding site of G85R SOD1 [36], resveratrol[38], natural polyphenols like curcumin, kaempferol, and kaempferideas possible lead drugs for the management of ALS [39].

Huntington's Disease (HD)

HD is a rare, inherited condition that results in the gradual breakdown (degeneration) of nerve cells in the brain.4-Aminobutyrate aminotransferase

(ABAT) degrades gamma-aminobutyric acid (GABA), a key inhibitory modulator of synaptic transmission in CNS.Many genetic abnormalities and chronic neurological disorders such as AD, PD, and HD cause a decrease in GABAergic transmission. Exogenous GABA cannot penetrate the BBB, thus it cannot be used directly [40]. An alternate method is to increase GABA levels by reducing its breakdown by ABAT. The structures of 32 compounds from 31 medicinal herbs were collected from a chemical database, and these 32 compounds were evaluated in a molecular docking analysis, with the top-ranked compounds being recommended for in vitro and in vivo investigations of ABAT inhibition [41].

Conclusion

In conclusion, we can bring to a close that the drug design and discovery process-based analysis of data will be a next-generation for computational neuroscience, and neuroinformatics, as well as reasonable approaches in software tools and resources. The approach will be a basement for the future treatment of diseases like PD, ALS, HD, and AD. The new branches like Computational Neurosciences and Neuroinformatics, Neuroscience databases, and tools will be new needles in a haystack to discover new regimens or treatments for neurological disorders.

References

[1] Stiles J. *The fundamentals of brain development: integrating nature and nurture;* Harvard University Press: 2008.

[2] Linne ML. Neuroinformatics and computational modelling as complementary tools for neurotoxicology studies. *Basic & Clinical Pharmacology & Toxicology,* 2018, 123, 56-61.

[3] Azevedo FA, Carvalho LR, Grinberg LT, Farfel JM, Ferretti RE, Leite RE, Filho WJ, Lent R, Herculano-Houzel S. Equal numbers of neuronal and nonneuronal cells make the human brain an isometrically scaled-up primate brain. *Journal of Comparative Neurology,* 2009, 513, 532-541.

[4] Kiernan MC. *A Fine Neuroscience Vintage*. BMJ Publishing Group Ltd: 2015.

[5] Copeland BJ, Shagrir O. Physical computation: How general are Gandy's principles for mechanisms? *Minds and Machines*, 2007, 17, 217-231.

[6] Piccinini G, Bahar S. Neural computation and the computational theory of cognition. *Cognitive Science*, 2013, 37, 453-488.

[7] Young MP, Scannell JW. Brain structure–function relationships: advances from neuroinformatics. *Philosophical Transactions of the Royal Society of London. Series B: Biological Sciences*, 2000, 355, 3-6.

[8] Nayak L, Dasgupta A, Das R, Ghosh K, De Rajat K. Computational neuroscience and neuroinformatics: recent progress and resources. *J Biosci*, 2018, 43, 1037-1054.

[9] Nayak L, Dasgupta A, Das R, Ghosh K, De RK. Computational neuroscience and neuroinformatics: recent progress and resources. *J Biosci,* 2018, 43, 1037-1054.

[10] Kriegeskorte N, Douglas PK. Cognitive computational neuroscience. *Nature Neuroscience*, 2018, 21, 1148-1160, doi:10.1038/s41593-018-0210-5.

[11] Bota M, Dong HW, Swanson LW. From gene networks to brain networks. *Nature Neuroscience*, 2003, 6, 795-799, doi:10.1038/nn1096.

[12] Kötter R. Neuroscience databases: tools for exploring brain structure-function relationships. *Philosophical Transactions of the Royal Society of London. Series B, Biological Sciences*, 2001, 356, 1111-1120, doi:10.1098/rstb.2001.0902.

[13] Teeters JL, Harris, KD, Millman KJ, Olshausen BA, Sommer FT. Data sharing for computational neuroscience. *Neuroinformatics,* 2008, 6, 47-55.

[14] Hassan Baig M, Ahmad K, Roy S, Mohammad Ashraf J, Adil M, Haris Siddiqui M, Khan S, Amjad Kamal M, Provazník I, Choi I. Computer aided drug design: success and limitations. *Current Pharmaceutical Design*, 2016, 22, 572-581.

[15] Macalino SJ, Gosu V, Hong S, Choi S. Role of computer-aided drug design in modern drug discovery. *Arch Pharm Res,* 2015, 38, 1686-1701, doi:10.1007/s122 72-015-0640-5.

[16] Khan S, Ahmad K, Alshammari E, Adnan M, Baig MH, Lohani M, Somvanshi P, Haque S. Implication of caspase-3 as a common therapeutic target for multineurodegenerative disorders and its inhibition using nonpeptidyl natural compounds. *BioMed Research International,* 2015, 2015.

[17] Krivanek TJ, Gale SA, McFeeley BM, Nicastri CM, Daffner KR. Promoting Successful Cognitive Aging: A Ten-Year Update. *Journal of Alzheimer's Disease,* 2021, 1-50.

[18] Baig MH, Ahmad K, Rabbani G, Danishuddin M, Choi I. Computer aided drug design and its application to the development of potential drugs for neurodegenerative disorders. *Current Neuropharmacology*, 2018, 16, 740-748.

[19] Ahmad K, Balaramnavar VM, Chaturvedi N, Khan S, Haque S, Lee Y-H, Choi I. Targeting Caspase 8: Using structural and ligand-based approaches to identify potential leads for the treatment of multi-neurodegenerative diseases. *Molecules,* 2019, 24, 1827.

[20] Ahmad K, Baig MH, Gupta GK, Kamal M, Pathak N, Choi I. Identification of common therapeutic targets for selected neurodegenerative disorders: an in silico approach. *Journal of Computational Science*, 2016, 17, 292-306.

[21] Gupta A, Bhunia S, Balaramnavar V, Saxena A. Pharmacophore modelling, molecular docking and virtual screening for EGFR (HER 1) tyrosine kinase inhibitors. *SAR and QSAR in Environmental Research,* 2011, 22, 239-263.

[22] Saxena A, Balaramnavar VM, Hohlfeld T, Saxena AK. Drug/drug interaction of common NSAIDs with antiplatelet effect of aspirin in human platelets. *European Journal of Pharmacology*, 2013, 721, 215-224.

[23] Chen D, Martin ZS, Soto C, Schein CH. Computational selection of inhibitors of a beta aggregation and neuronal toxicity. *Bioorg Med Chem,* 2009, 17, 5189-5197, doi:10.1016/j.bmc.2009.05.047.

[24] Fu H, Li W, Luo J, Lee NT, Li M, Tsim KW, Pang Y, Youdim MB, Han Y. Promising anti-Alzheimer's dimer bis(7)-tacrine reduces beta-amyloid generation by directly inhibiting BACE-1 activity. *Biochem Biophys Res Commun,* 2008, 366, 631-636, doi:10.1016/j.bbrc.2007.11.068.

[25] Jiang Y, Mullaney KA, Peterhoff CM, Che S, Schmidt SD, Boyer-Boiteau A, Ginsberg SD, Cataldo AM, Mathews PM, Nixon RA. Alzheimer's-related endosome dysfunction in Down syndrome is Abeta-independent but requires APP and is reversed by BACE-1 inhibition. *Proc Natl Acad Sci USA,* 2010, 107, 1630-1635, doi:10.1073/pnas.0908953107.

[26] Ju Y, Li Z, Deng Y, Tong A, Zhou L, Luo Y. Identification of Novel BACE1 Inhibitors by Combination of Pharmacophore Modeling, Structure-Based Design and In Vitro Assay. *Curr Comput Aided Drug Des,* 2016, 12, 73-82, doi:10.2174/1573409912666160222113103.

[27] Labandeira-Garcia JL, Rodriguez-Perez AI, Villar-Cheda B, Borrajo A, Dominguez-Meijide A, Guerra MJ. Rho Kinase and Dopaminergic Degeneration: A Promising Therapeutic Target for Parkinson's Disease. *Neuroscientist,* 2015, 21, 616-629, doi:10.1177/1073858414554954.

[28] Nayernia Z, Jaquet V, Krause KH. New insights on NOX enzymes in the central nervous system. *Antioxid Redox Signal,* 2014, 20, 2815-2837, doi:10.1089/ars.2013.5703.

[29] Alokam R, Singhal S, Srivathsav GS, Garigipati S, Puppala S, Sriram D, Perumal Y. Design of dual inhibitors of ROCK-I and NOX2 as potential leads for the treatment of neuroinflammation associated with various neurological diseases including autism spectrum disorder. *Mol Biosyst,* 2015, 11, 607-617, doi:10.1039/c4mb00570h.

[30] Tang H, Song P, Li J, Zhao D. Effect of Salvia miltiorrhiza on acetylcholinesterase: Enzyme kinetics and interaction mechanism merging with molecular docking analysis. *Int J Biol Macromol*, 2019, 135, 303-313, doi:10.1016/j.ijbiomac.2019.05.132.

[31] Ram H, Jaipal N, Kumar P, Deka P, Kumar S, Kashyap P, Kumar S, Singh BP, Alqarawi AA, Hashem A, et al. Dual Inhibition of DPP-4 and Cholinesterase Enzymes by the Phytoconstituents of the Ethanolic Extract of Prosopis cineraria Pods: Therapeutic Implications for the Treatment of Diabetes-associated Neurological Impairments. *Curr Alzheimer Res,* 2019, 16, 1230-1244, doi:10.2174/1567205016666191203161509.

[32] Sturchio A, Marsili L, Mahajan A, Grimberg MB, Kauffman MA, Espay AJ. How have advances in genetic technology modified movement disorder nosology? *Eur J Neurol*, 2020, 27, 1461-1470, doi:10.1111/ene.14294.

[33] Paul DA, Qureshi ARM, Rana AQ. Peripheral neuropathy in Parkinson's disease. *Neurol Sci,* 2020, 41, 2691-2701, doi:10.1007/s10072-020-04407-4.

[34] Ma Z, Liu H, Wu B. Structure-based drug design of catechol-O-methyltransferase inhibitors for CNS disorders. *Br J Clin Pharmacol,* 2014, 77, 410-420, doi:10.1111/bcp.12169.

[35] Wijesekera LC, Leigh PN. Amyotrophic lateral sclerosis. *Orphanet J Rare Dis,* 2009, 4, 3, doi:10.1186/1750-1172-4-3.

[36] Hirayama K, Fujiwara Y, Terada T, Shimizu K, Wada K, Kabuta T. Virtual screening identification of novel chemical inhibitors for aberrant interactions between pathogenic mutant SOD1 and tubulin. *Neurochem Int,* 2019, 126, 19-26, doi:10.1016/j.neuint.2019.02.020.

[37] Srinivasan E, Rajasekaran R. Rational design of linear tripeptides against the aggregation of human mutant SOD1 protein causing amyotrophic lateral sclerosis. *J Neurol Sci,* 2019, 405, 116425, doi:10.1016/j.jns.2019.116425.

[38] Srinivasan E, Rajasekaran R. Quantum chemical and molecular mechanics studies on the assessment of interactions between resveratrol and mutant SOD1 (G93A) protein. *J Comput Aided Mol Des,* 2018, 32, 1347-1361, doi:10.1007/s10822-018-0175-1.

[39] Srinivasan E, Rajasekaran R. Comparative binding of kaempferol and kaempferide on inhibiting the aggregate formation of mutant (G85R) SOD1 protein in familial amyotrophic lateral sclerosis: A quantum chemical and molecular mechanics study. *Biofactors,* 2018, 44, 431-442, doi:10.1002/ biof.1441.

[40] Boonstra E, de Kleijn R, Colzato LS, Alkemade A, Forstmann BU, Nieuwenhuis S. Neurotransmitters as food supplements: the effects of GABA on brain and behavior. *Front Psychol,* 2015, 6, 1520, doi:10.3389/ fpsyg.2015.01520.

[41] Vijayakumar S, Kasthuri G, Prabhu S, Manogar P, Parameswari N. Screening and identification of novel inhibitors against human 4-aminobutyrate-aminotransferase: a computational approach. *Egyptian Journal of Basic and Applied Sciences,* 2018, 5, 210-219.

Chapter 2

Neuroinformatics: Emerging Trends of Bioinformatics in Neuroscience

Aishwarya Banerjee, Arunima SenGupta, Haritha K. Haridas and Neetu Jabalia*

Amity Institute of Biotechnology, Amity University Uttar Pradesh, India

Abstract

Neuroscience is an ironic foundation of computational and informatics glitches. These issues include many applications of traditional bioinformatics to the neuroscience domain. Bioinformatics has been an accelerating growth area in the past few years. Neuroinformatics combines neuroscience with biological science with information technology and aids in dealing with the production and maintenance of web applications that will be required to achieve such integration. Hence, one of the objectives of this chapter is to present a comprehensive overview on bioinformatics, neuroscience and neuroinformatics. In other words, snapshot of bioinformatics to understand its impact on neurogenomics. The latter dimension describes databases of neuroinformatics and their applications. The last part of this chapter discusses bioinformatics and in silico modelling in the field of Neuroscience that will assist the readers in utilizing the data to their best advantage.

Keywords: bioinformatics, neuroinformatics, neurosciences, database

---

* Corresponding Author Email: njabalia@gmail.com.

In: New Perspectives in Neuroscience
Editors: Prachi Srivastava, Neha Srivastava and Prekshi Garg
ISBN: 978-1-68507-754-9

Introduction

As one of the most complicated organs of the human body, neuroscience is primarily focused on understanding the development, function, organization and the structure of the nervous system, irrespective of the brain being healthy or diseased. Essentially, Neuroinformatics combines neuroscience and information technology, or to put it differently, an area of applied knowledge that focuses on the building and maintenance of data sets and databases that make it easy for people to access through the use of information resources. Beginning in the mid-1900s, neuroinformatics endeavoured to understand the CNS in a healthy state as well as in the event of a disorder. The resulting decade saw a betterment which was inclusive of the management of the complicated data that is needed in the middle of the clinical study pertaining to the nervous system. Researchers from EMBL and GenBank, two banks operated by the European Molecular Biology research facility, began dispatching data sets to each other in the mid-1980s.

Neuroinformatics is defined as an arena that profits from cumulative cooperative energies among neuroscience and data innovation, for example, manages the use of cutting edge Information technology (IT) techniques to manage the surge of neuroscientific information by creating and applying information investigation strategies for the investigation of the mind; by giving both logical and mathematical instruments for hypothetically demonstrating cerebrum work; and by abusing our experiences into the standards hidden mind capacity to foster new IT advancements. Researchers have examined the brain utilizing different strategies, including magnetic resonance imaging (MRI), functional magnetic resonance imaging (fMRI), and computed tomography (CT), to consider the capacity, availability, and construction of the brain; microarray analysis., in situ hybridization (ISH) and next generation sequencing (NGS) to examine the atomic condition of the mind; electroencephalography (EEG) and magnetoencephalography (MEG) to contemplate the electrophysiology of the brain. Along these lines, neuroscience has become vital for the neuroscience agents and clinicians for directing logical requests, understanding the reason and pathogenesis of a mind issue and rehearsing medication [1].

As a practical matter, bioinformatics entails scrutinizing as well as analysing and storing genomes (DNA), related particles (RNA, proteins), and, in addition, displaying the structural and functional characteristics of both existing and new (planned) proteins that the blast of action in bioinformatics has developed past the beginning of bioinformatics. In general, bioinformatics can be described as a synthesis of science (life sciences) and informatics (PC and measurable techniques). Figure 1 depicts the framework of bioinformatics in neuroscience [2].

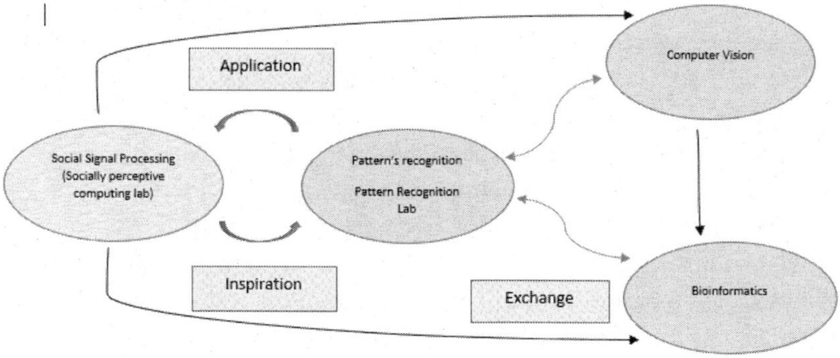

Figure 1. Flowchart representing bioinformatics and neuroscience.

Bioinformatics

The fast-proliferating field of computational biology or in other words bioinformatics encompasses mathematics, essentials of biology along with information science and aids in answering queries pertaining to biology. The term 'bioinformatics' was coined in the year of 1968 and the term was bestowed with a proper description in the year 1978. Bioinformatics is also widely known as computational biology. But fundamentally, computational biology refers to the creation of artificial biological models using various tools. The science of bioinformatics is comprised of two major parts, the first being, the creation of algorithms and tools for using software and the other being, the use of different tools of software and specific algorithms for the study and elucidation of biological data [3]. Genetics, biology and medicine have all become engrossed with computational biology, which has become more and more exciting. We can even consider Bioinformatics as a concept that encompasses all the primary functions of information 9 technology in the molecular biology area [4].

In the biological analysis of recent times, bioinformatics research plays an important factor. An integral part of the biology of the constantly expanding biological database is bioinformatics, a multidisciplinary area within the spectrum of life sciences which combines mathematical and computer science approaches. Biological data is accessed by creating methods and analytical tools to understand, analyse, extract, store, organize, systemize, annotate, visualize, mine, and interpret the exponential amounts of data available [5]. The primary database of computational biology is inclusive of sequences of genes as well as complete genomes which comprises proteins made up of amino acid sequences, three-dimensional protein formations and nucleic acid complexes made up of nucleic acids as well as proteins. Data associated with "-omics" has been collected on the following subjects: protein disintegration within cells, transcriptomics, proteomics, interactomics, metabolomics, RNA development from DNA, protein-protein interactions, and the nature of 10 molecule changing by biochemical mechanisms within cells.

There is an augmented intrigue towards the obtainment of understandable, articulate and precise data for certain types of cells, also towards the identification of motifs of modifications within the databases and datasets in every possible case. For instance, there can be variance in data depending upon the type of cell, the time of aggregation of data in the midst of the cell cycle or in the middle of seasonal, annual or diurnal diversifications, during the stage of development as well as varied outward conditions. Measurements like these are augmented to a more exhaustive definition of living organisms within a natural sample vis-à-vis in a container of oceanic water or in a sample of soil by bringing to use meta proteomics as well as metagenomics. The prompt development in the processes pertaining to generation of data in the field of biology primarily drives bioinformatics. The most striking effects is seen as a result of approaches pertaining to genome sequencing. The archives of sequences of nucleic acids comprised nucleotides that amounted up to 3.5 billion in totality which turns out to be a little more than the expanse of a singular human genome in 1999. In 2009, the number of nucleotides increased to more than 283 billion which amounts to about ninety-five human genomic lengths.

Augmenting of experimental information through predictions is the main aim of computational biology. Another primary aim of bioinformatics is the prognosis of the structure of a protein sequence by analysing the sequence of amino acids. The possibility of this is depicted through the instinctive protein folding. CASP programs also known as Critical Assessment of Structure Prediction programs biennially measures the advancement in the growth of approaches for the prognosis of folding of proteins which is inclusive of blind examinations structure prognosis approaches.

Computational biology is also used as a prognostic approach for the prediction of interactions amid varied proteins after knowledge of the separate structures of these proteins. This is referred to as the docking problem. The shape of the surfaces along with the polarity of complexes that are protein-protein in nature depict brilliant complementarity. They are further made stable by interactions that are weak, embedding of the surface that is hydrophobic, H-bonds as well as Van derwaals forces. Software's work towards the simulation of such bond interactions towards the prognosis of proper spatial interaction amid two binding entities. A specific hurdle that needs to be overcome is to be able to create an antibody that aids in binding using a higher affinity to the protein body that forms the target. This challenge if overcome would prove to be of humongous therapeutic application. Most of the studies pertaining to bioinformatics, in the beginning had a very minute aim of concentrating completely on algorithm creation for the analysis of specific kinds of data, like sequences of genes or structures of proteins. In recent times, the aims of bioinformatics have shifted towards a more integrative approach and work towards finding out how a blend of varied kinds of brain data could be utilized to comprehend phenomena that are natural, inclusive of various organisms as well as disorders. [6]. Figure 2 shows the data utilized for neuroscience by implementing various bioinformatics applications.

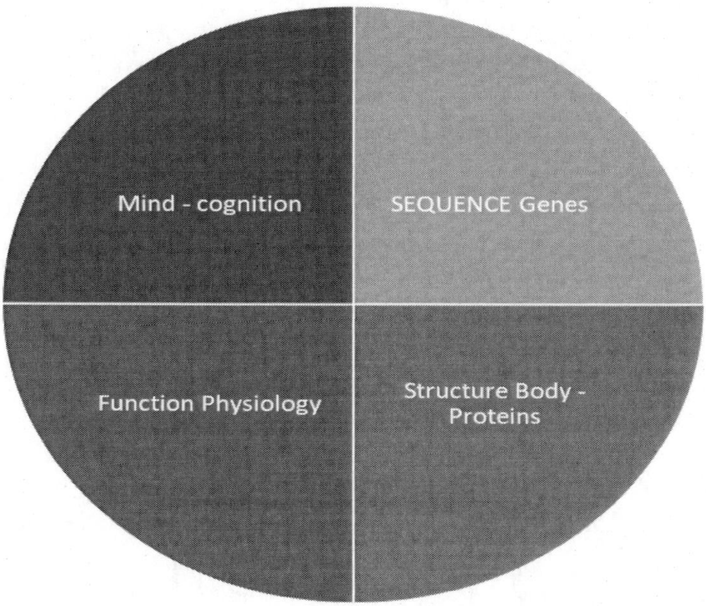

Figure 2. Development process of bioinformatics in neuroscience.

Neuroinformatics

Neuroscience forms a humongous pool of intriguing issues that are largely computational as well as associate to informatics. A lot of predictable bioinformatics is covered by these problems related to the area of neuroscience, for instance, analysis of gene sequences. Additionally, the term neuroinformatics came into play because the field of neuroscience has seen major application of computation and bioinformatics in comparison to other fields for the varied issues specific to the domain. Database creation of various standards, bioinformatics tools and models, replication construction, and analytic methodologies for the entire nervous system framework. In neuroinformatics where there is a requirement of extensive analysis of the sequence of gene and proteins, an extensive overlapping is usually found with the essentialities of conventional bioinformatics. Most of the interest in the field of neuroinformatics is brought about by the existence of the varied kinds of studies pertaining to neuroscience in addition to their association with more precision by bring to use the tools used in information technology [7].

Neuroinformatics endows the primary aim of conceptualizing the role of the various brain functions in the arena of health and disorders. This is inclusive of effective investigation of various stages of interactions that are complex occurring within the folds of cellular biology, the global brain networks, cortical microcircuits and cognitive mechanisms. For being able to get past this aim, it is essential to develop huge databases wherein it is plausible to share a plethora of uniform, data related to neuroscience, development of strong tools for the purpose of investigation along with the creation of models for accurate computation. The above mentioned three requirements form the backbone of what neuroinformatics essentially focusses on [8].

A large number of approaches have been created to augment the amount of research in the arena of bioinformatics pertaining to neuroscience. The most notable of these approaches is the Human Brain Project or in other words the HBP, which also was the first of such approaches initiated in the year of 1993. A huge number of projects in the arena of neuroinformatics received proper guidance as well as funding from the Human Brain Project under the aegis of National Institute of Mental Health as well as several others (National Institute of Homeopathy) NIH institutes. The NIH Blueprint for Neuroscience research formed the successor of the Human Brain Project as the field of neuroinformatics has been seeing huge integration into the major fields of neuroscience along with informatics. In case of resource development for generalised use towards the studies in the field of neuroscience, Blueprint for Neuroscience research was brought forth as a huge cumulative initiative. The major focus of informatics in the field of neuroscience can also be gauged by the point that the newly created International Neuroinformatics Coordinating Facility abbreviated (INCF), which is funded by the European Union and is based out of Stockholm, Sweden, having nodes across a multitude of European countries in addition to its nodes being spread across US as well as Japan has set aside a goal to restore and retain international interest in the arena of neuroinformatics. In accordance to a report by Organization for Economic Co-operation and Development (OECD), the INCF came into emergence.

The task force of the Brain Information Group was brought together in the year of 2003 by the Society for Neuroscience (SfN) which was later prospered by the SfN Neuroinformatics committee. These groups and committees were started to scrutinize the requirements of informatics in the field of neuroscience and is also aimed at the continued promotion of remaining resources [10]. Neuroscience database (NDB) gateway substantiated as the best consequence. A total of 178 databases are neatly arranged into five major categories and a whole of fifteen classes by the Neuroscience database gateway. The Neuroscience Information Framework stands as NDB's successor through persistent cumulative efforts. In the phase of research and exploration, this agenda is considered to provide easy access through links to databases, tools along with other results, organised and clarified by bringing to use a formally controlled vocabulary known as the BrainML (Brain Markup Language).

The BIRN or Biomedical Informatics Research Network backed up by the NIH, is a project on a huge scale largely known for the scale along with its scope when it comes to the fields of neuroscience and informatics. BIRN focusses mainly on neuroinformatics and puts major emphasis on the brain imaging of essentially human beings and mice. In case of primary and medical research, BIRN also emphasizes on hardware creation, software and protocols for proper sharing and mining data in a more site independent manner. BIRN makes use of work being conducted in about 12 laboratories spread across the USA as well as the UK [9].

Computational neuroscience can be largely referred to as the systems biology of neuroscience and essentially involves the creation and subsequent application of bioinformatics models of the nervous system as well as their other constituents. There is a plethora of resources that further work towards creation of models pertaining to single neurons, sensory processing, information processing and networks. A more focused form of the research is inclusive of a study of the functioning memory; sensorimotor changes object identification as well as visual attention. Top-down and bottom-up are the categories given to modelling approaches. In the approach that is bottom-up, deeply analysed information of the system, for instance, neuronal network is utilized in the creation of a model. Likewise, in case of top-down approaches, the systems inputs as well as outputs are considered first, for instance, a firing motif involving the behaviour and neurons to interpret strategies for proper computation that the system working behind this may bring to use. Both of the two methods are meant to create hypotheses that can be tested pertaining to the working of the neuronal systems.

We possess very minute knowledge of the systems which hinders our capability to model and understand nervous systems, especially when it comes to the approach that is bottom-up. Very few neuronal systems are present that can be comprehended at that level, leading to a continued expectation in the systems biology study of the networks of the biochemical pathways. The continued effort to incorporate omics into the field of neuroscience is supposed to create a huge impact. Computational biology includes the enhanced approaches of computer software's to evaluate and comprehend various issues in the medical as well as biological field. The functioning of bioinformatics in the area of neurosciences is known as neuroinformatics or in other words NI. The field of biomedicine underwent major evolvement due to databases, data mining along with modelling of data. The Human Genome Project (HGP) is the primary undertaking pertaining to computational biology. Each and every area of neuroscience has witnessed some chief revolutions because of the rise of bioinformatics. However, the arena of neuroinformatics is yet to be properly explored in the area of neuropsychology. Neuro-informatics has to offer huge amount of potential to the field of neuropsychology through proper gauging of cognitive behaviour and drawing a relation between the cognitive abilities along with the neural systems [10].

During the initial phase of the 1990's utilization of neuroinformatics as an area primarily aimed at the establishment of databases along with comprehension tools for the nervous system was brought into emergence. In the following decade, enhancement was initiated towards working with complicated data types that pertained to the examination of nervous system. To deal with the constantly increasing number of databases as well as tools certain websites or databases are required. SfN in 2004 and Neuroscience Database Gateway in 2007 were brought into emergence to cut across this challenge, after which a more enhanced framework known as the Neuroscience Information Framework 2007 proved to be more fruitful [11].

The understanding of the complicated arena of neuroinformatics can be eased out by initially comprehending the associated field of bioinformatics. During the latter part of 1970's the initial collections of the data of proteins were done. Research analysts understood that to keep a tab on the letter sequence for instance GCAT that shaped the base sequence representation that is involved in the creation of nucleic acids or the sequence of amino acids that are behind the making up of proteins, computer is an essentiality. In the initial part of 1980s, European Molecular Biology laboratory's EMBL-Bank, National Centre for Biotechnology along with Databases for genes, were brought into emergence [12].

The field of neuroscience and the biomedical field is supported by a pool of databases as well as tools pertaining to neuroscience (Figure 3). An augmented version of tools that are analogous in nature than those found before can be perceived as the field of neuroinformatics. The various parts of neuroscience data are starting to be organised using databases within databases. Assessment and modelling of nervous systems at scales that are more spatial could be done through neuroinformatics [13].

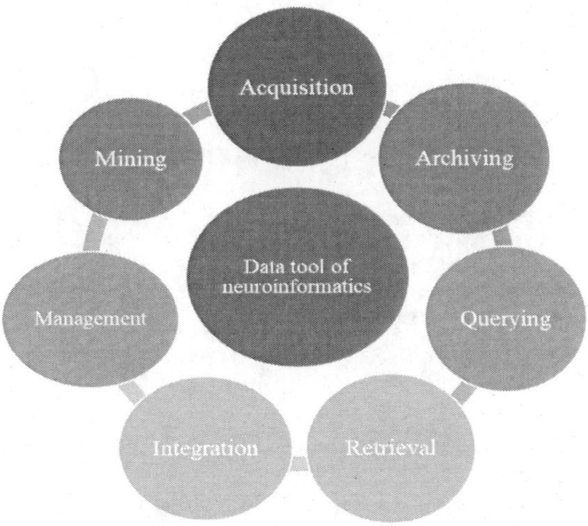

Figure 3. Data tools of neuroinformatics.

Neurogenomics

There have been a huge number of contributions made towards enhancing our conceptualization of the functioning, development as well as the evolution of the nervous system, along with the variance found within species as well as the diversity in them through recent and innovative genomic techniques. Although, majority of these advancements in research have been part of nations that have modern and enhanced scientific resources and firm and reliable support systems for funds. In contrast, not much is known about the plausible interaction amid varied genetic factors, elements that are non-coding in nature along with environmental aspects in analysing disorders pertaining to neurology amid the people belonging to countries which are not very rich which particularly is inclusive of a multitude of African countries. Populations indigenous to Africa possess a one-of-a-kind ancestry which brings to light that the betterment in the inclusion of people from this area in gene analysis that are associated to neuroscience would largely aid in the acknowledgment of first-hand and innovative factors which will help in the development of the future of the field of neuroscience and healthcare pertaining to neurology.

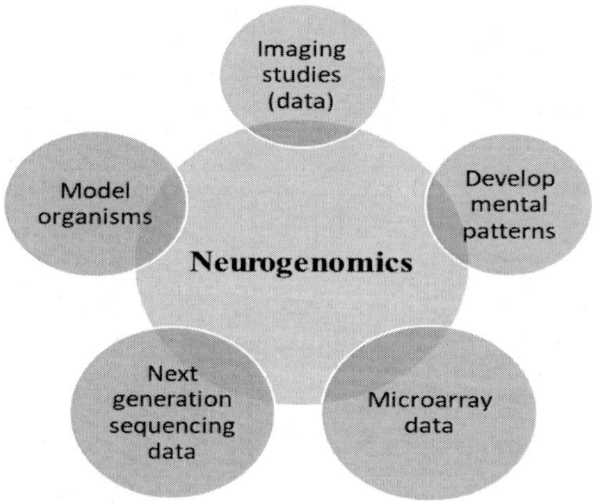

Figure 4. Areas of focus in neurogenomics.

This assumption is hugely backed up by the latest finding which points that patient with disorders and their respective kins from certain populations belonging to the sub-Saharan Africa do not possess the specific gene mutations associated to the neurological disorders. This suggests that certain neurological illnesses may be linked to population specificity, highlighting the need for more research into the role of other currently unidentified genetic variables [14]. Figure 4 shows the systemic representation of focused areas of neurogenomics.

Database for Neuroinformatics

During the ensuing decade improvement began on managing the unpredictable sorts of information that describe investigations of the sensory system. Neuroinformatics compile web-available data sets of trial and computational information, along with inventive programming apparatuses, which is basic for comprehending the nervous system in its ordinary capacity and in neurological issues. Neuroinformatics incorporates conventional bioinformatics of quality and protein groupings in the mind; map books of cerebrum life systems and confinement of qualities and protein molecules; imaging and recognition of synapses; mind imaging done through positron discharge tomography (PET), functional magnetic resonance imaging(fMRI), electroencephalography (EEG), magnetoencephalography (MEG) and different strategies; numerous electrophysiological recording techniques; and clinical neurological information, among others. Building neuroinformatics information bases and instruments presents troublesome difficulties since they length a wide scope of spatial scales and sorts of information put away and dissected. Conventional bioinformatics, by examination, centres fundamentally around genomic and proteomic information (which obviously likewise presents troublesome difficulties). A lot of bioinformatics investigation centre around arrangements (DNA, RNA, as well as protein atomic bodies), as the kind of information which have been put away, analysed, and once in a while displayed. Bioinformatics is going through unstable development with the expansion, for instance, of data sets that inventory associations between proteins, of data sets that track the advancement of qualities, and of frameworks science data sets which is inclusive of prototypes of all parts of creatures.

Neuroinformatics exploratory information bases may store capacity and life structures explanations of sensory system qualities, pictures (procured with various strategies, for example, primary as well as functional magnetic resonance imaging (MRI as well as fMRI respectively), staining of tissues at spatial scales from subcellular electron magnifying instrument pictures to many centimetres cuts however brains of monkeys, optical accounts of voltage and synthetic actuated colours, so on and so forth), and chart books of focal and fringe sensory systems. A few activities handled the troublesome issue of open finished information offering to heterogeneous information [15-18]. Exploratory and unmistakable data, in the open finished case, has been reported with meta-information which depicts its substance and configuration for effective sharing. Different ventures endeavoured to progress new exploratory strategies (wavelet investigation in fMRI [19] and information examination instruments for MRI planning of cerebrums to surfaces for correlation between minds from similar species (in people this has clinical applications, and furthermore correlations between various species sensory systems [20]. Further devices permit the acknowledgment of items inside the fMRI informational indexes, improve the nature of fMRI pictures and frameworks to store and share fMRI informational collections. Different undertakings were intended to arrangement data sets of in-situ hybridization information to give a perpetual available file to assets at risk for vanishing (a lot of this information exists in slides in singular examiners research centres) (Interactive y Multiple Gene Expression Maps 2008). A few activities made online map books and guides of human, macaque (monkey), rodent, and mouse cerebrums (see information bases having chart books as classes in SfN Neuroscience Database Gateway 2007). A few tasks consolidated data sets of pictures with explanations of quality articulation.

Hypothetical neuroinformatics projects handled assorted subjects: displaying cortical guides, putting on display the olfactory bulb and putting away models based on computational neuroscience in a web available information base, growing new wavelet based and source partition examination apparatuses for fMRI information, itemized devices for neuromorphological displaying, programmed cortical surface remaking planning and instruments for indicating a 2-D arrange framework for the planning, and making sensible computational models equipped for anticipating human hear-able reactions to a wide scope of acoustic boosts including acoustic injury. There is a wide assortment of neuroscience information bases and devices that help neuroscience and biomedicine. The field of neuroinformatics may be witnessed as an all-including and expounded use of closely resembling apparatuses to those discovered before to be basic for the advancement of bioinformatics, however applied to a more extensive, heterogeneous sorts of information at numerous degrees of capacity. The profundity and broadness of neuroscience data is starting to be coordinated through data sets of information bases. These, and the data in the information bases they contain, will help looking in, contrasting, and displaying sensory systems at spatial scales from the degree of atoms to conduct, in typical, unhealthy, or harmed people and creatures. Neuroinformatics is getting crucial for neuroscience agents and clinicians for leading logical request, and rehearsing medication presently of quickly growing cross-disciplinary information [21].

National Centre for Biotechnology Information (NCBI)

A neuroscience search that exhibits a cover in customary bioinformatics and neuroinformatics begins with an "All data set" search at PubMed (National Centre for Biotechnology Information 2007). This amazing web index at the same time look through 28 data sets which remembers sections for the assorted subjects of writing (articles in diaries and books), grouping data or information bases and metadata (depictions of the information or organization in which the information is put away), data sets on Journals (themselves, not the articles in them) and jargon, and bibliographic information pertaining to the National Library of Medicine property of books, programming, and different assets. This is valuable to at the same time discover data about qualities and furthermore the writing that depicts discoveries about the quality. An inquiry on the Parkinson's connected quality PINK1 brings about 114 articles found in PubMed, anyway utilizing the Medical Subject Heading (MeSH) (National Library of Medicine 2007) terms (chose "significant words," for example words whose definitions are unequivocally indicated, the hunt "PINK1 AND PARKINSON'S[MeSH]" discovers 67 articles which are then known to be pertinent to PARKINSON'S sickness. The MeSH expressions aids the client in discovering the things in the sets of data that have the right setting, for example the Nucleotide grouping information base (incorporates GenBank) discovers 41 hits in the unlimited PINK1 search, notwithstanding, when the PARKINSON'S expression is added the quantity of hits drops to 2 and the reports related with the passages are focused on to Parkinson's clinical exploration. This model exhibited how designated look through an assortment of data sets produces outcomes that are of quick premium to the agent of neuroscience [22].

Neuroscience Database Gateway (NDG)

Permit us to visualize that we are a specialist hunting for sites that contain human cerebrum map books to rethink some aspect of sensory system life structures. Beginning at the NDG (SfN Neuroscience Database Gateway 2007) landing page click on the "Search" interface in the left-hand section and enter "Map book" under classifications and "Human" under species and press the "Search" button. In the event that the hunt terms are not known the "watchword" catches for each field can be squeezed which spring up a window where numerous pursuit terms can be chosen [23].

Table 1. List of in-silico applications for neuroinformatics

S. No	Database/Web server	Description	Link
1	Brain-imaging database	Brain imaging is divided into mainly two different areas, structural imaging technique and functional imaging techniques	https://www.oasis-brains.org/
2	Brain-development.org	It contains datasets of over 600 Magnetic Resonance Imaging images of healthy subjects which utilizes Tissue 1 Tissue 2 and PD weighted images.	https://brain-development.org/
3	Brainmuseum.org	It is a public web site that provides the images and the information of well preserved, sectioned and stained brains of over 100 species of mammals including humans.	http://www.brainmuseum.org/
4	Harvard whole brain atlas	It contains a huge compilation of modern cross sectional signaling including CT (Computed tomography), MRI (magnetic resonance imaging) and SPECT (single photon emission computerized tomography) in health and diseased condition of brains.	https://www.med.harvard.edu/aanlib/home.html
5	Brainmap.org	It involves the development of software and tools to share neuroimaging results and enable meta-analysis of studies of human brain function and structure in healthy and diseased subjects.	https://www.brainmap.org/
6	Brainmaps.org	It is an interactive multiresolution next generation brain atlas that is based on over 20 million megapixels of submicron resolution, annotated, scanned images of serial sections of both primates, and non-primate brain,	http://brainmaps.org/
7	Neuromorpho.org	It is the largest public repository of 3- D digital neuronal reconstruction and associated metadata.it can be used for analysis, visualization and modelling of neuronal data.	http://neuromorpho.org/
8	NeuroElectro	It is a database describing the electrophysiology properties of different neuron types to understand the role of diversity across neuron types.	https://neuroelectro.org/
9	Code Analysis, Modelling and Repository for E-Neuroscience (CARMEN) Project	It provides a web-based portal platform through which users can share and collaboratively exploit data	https://portal.carmen.org.uk

S. No	Database/Web server	Description	Link
10	Collaborative Research in Computational Neuroscience (CRNCS)	It provides a forum of discussion over electrophysiological datasets as well as involved in sharing data.	https://crcns.org/
11	Brain connectivity databases	It provides the neuroanatomical images and the ultimate aim is to reconstruct the 3D model of the brain.	https://www.nitrc.org/projects/cocomac/#:~:text=CoCoMac.org%20gives%20online%20access,four%20hundred%20published%20tracing%20studies.
12	CoCoMac	It is the main database and contains data from tracing studies on anatomical connectivity in the macaque cerebral cortex.	http://cocomac.g-node.org/main/index.php?
13	BAMS (Brain architecture management system)	It is an online database having the information about the neural circuitry, brain connectivity database and an ontology of brain regions.	https://bams1.org/
14	Databases for genetic information	Gene expressions in various brain regions and various cell types are important information for understanding a relationship between regulation of molecular level and physiological level of brains.	https://www.ncbi.nlm.nih.gov/gene/
15	SigCS base	It is an integrated genetic information resource for human cerebral stroke.	http://sysbio.kribb.re.kr/sigcs
16	Gene expression omnibus (GEO)	It provides a flexible and an open design that facilitate submission, storage and retrieval of heterogeneous data sets from gene expression and genomic hybridization experiments [26].	https://www.ncbi.nlm.nih.gov/geo/
17	ArrayExpress	It is a new public database of microarray gene expression data which is a generic gene expression database designed to hold data from all microarray platforms.	https://www.ebi.ac.uk/arrayexpress/
18	Allen brain atlas	Allen Human Brain Atlas provides gene expression from human whole brain regions which is the first and unique multi-modal gene expression atlas of the human brain.	https://portal.brain-map.org/

Neuroinformatics Database (NiDB)

NiDB was created at Hartford Hospital for the Olin Neuropsychiatry Research Centre to store and deal with various kinds of information investigations. NIDB is an incredible, simple to introduce neuroimaging data set intended to permit basic bringing in, looking, and sharing of imaging information. NIDB relates any methodology imaging or other parallel information (MR, CT, US, EEG, and so forth) with a subject through quite a few imaging studies or activities. Information is kept at your site, constrained by you, to be imparted to different locales at whatever point you need. NIDB likewise gives computerized pipelining bringing of results once more into NIDB which can be looked alongside imaging meta information [24, 25].

There are various other databases or web applications that can be used for neuroinformatics analysis (Table 1).

Conclusion

Bioinformatics is undergoing explosive advancements with the addition, of databases and web servers that catalogue interactions between proteins, of databases that track the evolution of genes, and of systems biology databases which contain models of all aspects of organisms. The understanding of the brain requires the development and application of suitable electronic tools to handle, represent, transform, analyze, and synthesize digital neuroscience data. In turn, such a challenge is the key solution to preventing, diagnosing, and treating brain diseases. Hence, neuroinformatics is a chief illustration of the current speeding up energizing development in traditional bioinformatics where data sets, are fundamental for understanding the sensory system in its ordinary capacity.

References

[1] Nayak, Losiana, Abhijit Dasgupta, Ritankar Das, Kuntal Ghosh, and Rajat K. De. 7 "Computational Neuroscience and Neuroinformatics: Recent Progress and Resources." *Journal of Biosciences* 43, no. 5 (2018): 1037-054. doi:10.1007/s12038-018-9813-y.

[2] Nielsen, Finn Årup. "Brede Tools and Federating Online Neuroinformatics Databases." 9 *Neuroinformatics* 12, no. 1 (2013): 27-37. doi:10.1007/s12021-013-9183-4.

[3] French, L., and P. Pavlidis. "Informatics in Neuroscience." *Briefings in Bioinformatics* 8, no. 6 (2007): 446-56. doi:10.1093/bib/bbm047.

[4] Luscombe, N. M., D. Greenbaum, and M. Gerstein. "What Is Bioinformatics? A Proposed Definition and Overview of the Field." *Methods of Information in Medicine* 40, no. 04 1 (2001): 346-58. doi:10.1055/s-0038-1634431.

[5] Milano, Marianna. "Gene Prioritization Tools." *Encyclopedia of Bioinformatics and Computational Biology*, 2019, 907-14. doi:10.1016/b978-0-12-809633-8.20406-8.

[6] Li, Jiajia, Ronald P. De Vries, and Mao Peng. "Bioinformatics Approaches for Fungal Biotechnology." *Encyclopedia of Mycology*, 2021, 536-54. doi:10.1 016/ b978-0-12- 819990-9.00012-3.

[7] Collier, James H., Lloyd Allison, Arthur M. Lesk, Peter J. Stuckey, Maria Garcia De La Banda, and Arun S. Konagurthu. "Statistical Inference of Protein Structural Alignments 34 Using Information and Compression." *Bioinformatics,* 2017. doi:10.1093/bioinformatics/btw757.

[8] Eisenhaber, Frank. *Discovering Biomolecular Mechanisms with Computational Biology*. Boston: Springer, 2006. doi:10.1007/0-387-36747-0.

[9] Eisenhaber, Frank. *"Prediction of Protein Function."* Discovering Biomolecular Mechanisms with Computational Biology Molecular Biology *Intelligence Unit*: 39-54. doi:10.1007/0-387-36747-0_4.

[10] Jagaroo, Vinoth. "Neuroinformatics for Neuropsychology." *Neuroinformatics for Neuropsychology*, 2009, 25-84. doi:10.1007/978-1-4419-0060-9_3.

[11] Morse, Thomas M. "Article Commentary: Neuroinformatics: From Bioinformatics to Databasing." *Bioinformatics and Biology Insights* 2, 2008 doi:10.4137/b bi.s540.

[12] Ouzounis, C. A., and A. Valencia. "Early Bioinformatics: The Birth of a Discipline-A Personal View." *Bioinformatics* 19, no. 17 (2003): 2176-190. doi:10.1093/bioi nformatics/btg309.

[13] Martone, Maryann E., Amarnath Gupta, and Mark H. Ellisman. "E-Neuroscience: Challenges and Triumphs in Integrating Distributed Data from Molecules to 5 Brains." *Nature Neuroscience* 7, no. 5 (2004): 467-72. doi:10.1038/nn1229.

[14] Karikari, Thomas K., and Jelena Aleksic. "Neurogenomics: An Opportunity to Integrate Neuroscience, Genomics and Bioinformatics Research in Africa." *Applied & Translational Genomics* 5 (2015): 3-10. doi:10.1016/j.atg.2015.06.004.

[15] Morse, Thomas M. "Article Commentary: Neuroinformatics: From Bioinformatics to Databasing the Brain." *Bioinformatics and Biology Insights* 2 (2008). doi:10.4137/bbi.s540.

[16] Gardner, D., K. H. Knuth, M. Abato, S. M. Erde, T. White, R. Debellis, and E. P. Gardner. "Common Data Model for Neuroscience Data and Data Model Exchange." *Journal of the American Medical Informatics Association* 8, 1 (2001): 17-33. doi:10.1136/jamia.2001.0080017.

[17] Lam, Hugo Yk, Luis Marenco, Tim Clark, Yong Gao, June Kinoshita, Gordon Shepherd, Perry Miller, Elizabeth Wu, Gwendolyn T. Wong, Nian Liu, Chiquito Crasto, Thomas Morse, Susie Stephens, and Kei-Hoi Cheung. "AlzPharm:

Integration of Neurodegeneration Data Using RDF." *BMC Bioinformatics* 8, no. Suppl 3 (2007). doi:10.1186/1471-2105-8-s3-s4.

[18] Marenco, Luis, Tzuu-Yi Wang, Gordon Shepherd, Perry L. Miller, and Prakash Nadkarni. "QIS: A Framework for Biomedical Database Federation." *Journal of the American Medical Informatics Association* 11, no. 6 (2004): 523-34. doi:10.1197/jamia.m1506.

[19] Martone, Maryann E., Amarnath Gupta, and Mark H. Ellisman. "E-Neuroscience: Challenges and Triumphs in Integrating Distributed Data from Molecules to Brains." *Nature Neuroscience* 7, no. 5 (2004): 467-72. doi:10.1038/nn1229.

[20] Fadili, M.j., and E.t. Bullmore. "Wavelet-Generalized Least Squares: A New BLU Estimator of Linear Regression Models with 1/f Errors." *NeuroImage* 15, no. 1 (2002): 217-32. doi:10.1006/nimg.2001.0955.

[21] Toga, Arthur W., Paul M. Thompson, Susumu Mori, Katrin Amunts, and Karl Zilles. "Towards Multimodal Atlases of the Human Brain." *Nature Reviews Neuroscience* 7, no. 12 (2006): 952-66. doi:10.1038/nrn2012.

[22] Morse, Thomas M. "Article Commentary: Neuroinformatics: From Bioinformatics to Databasing the Brain." *Bioinformatics and Biology Insights* 2 (2008). doi:10.4137/bbi.s540.

[23] Book, Gregory A., Beth M. Anderson, Michael C. Stevens, David C. Glahn, Michal Assaf, and Godfrey D. Pearlson. "Neuroinformatics Database (NiDB) – A Modular, Portable Database for the Storage, Analysis, and Sharing of Neuroimaging Data." *Neuroinformatics* 11, no. 4 (2013): 495-505. doi:10.1007/s12021-013-9194-1.

[24] "HUG 26 A, Ff. 082r-83v, Inc. 2a 2cc/(c A)." *Codices Hugeniani Online*. doi:10.1163/2468-0303-cohu_26a-046.

[25] Dmitri, Chklovskii. "Using Neuroinformatics Tools to Investigate and Share Highresolution Full Volume Reconstructions of Brain Neuropil." *Frontiers in Neuroinformatics* 2 (2008). doi:10.3389/conf.neuro.11.2008.01.155.

[26] Alawieh, Ali, Fadi A. Zaraket, Jian-Liang Li, Stefania Mondello, Amaly Nokkari, Mahdi Razafsha, Bilal Fadlallah, Rose-Mary Boustany, and Firas H. Kobeissy. "Systems Biology, Bioinformatics, and Biomarkers in Neuropsychiatry." *Frontiers in Neuroscience* 6 (2012). doi:10.3389/fnins.2012.00187.

Chapter 3

Neurotoxic Effects of Azo Food Colourants in Exposed Individuals

Pronit Biswas and Rajesh Singh Yadav*
Department of Criminology & Forensic Science, School of Applied Sciences (SAS), Dr. Harisingh Gour Vishwavidyalaya, A Central University, Sagar, MP, India

Abstract

Food products are artificially coloured to make attractive mixtures of basic ingredients of the food products to lure consumers. Food colourants are important food additives that enhanced the appearance of food and appetite. Studies suggested that azo food colourants cover about 65% of the total commercial market volume in the food colour industry and are injudiciously used in the food industry which imparts serious health risks to the exposed individual. The use of colourants in food products is subjected to a wide range of toxicity tests including acute, sub-chronic, chronic toxicity, carcinogenicity, mutagenicity and teratogenicity. Children are at a higher risk of toxicity as they consumed alluring food products such as cotton candy, soft drinks, flavoured chips, cereals, cake mixes, soups, sauces, ice cream, chewing gum, jam, jelly, etc. Studies have also suggested that exposure to these food colourants founded to be associated with the increased risk of attention deficit hyperactivity disorder (ADHD) and other motor dysfunctions in children. Keeping in view the exposure pattern of azo food colourants, the present book chapter is aimed to provide brief and systematic knowledge about the neurotoxicity induced by the azo food colourants in exposed individuals.

Keywords: food colourants, azo dyes, toxicity, neurotoxicity

---

*Corresponding Author's Email: razitrc@gmail.com.

In: New Perspectives in Neuroscience
Editors: Prachi Srivastava, Neha Srivastava and Prekshi Garg
ISBN: 978-1-68507-754-9

Introduction

The food colourants are any dye, pigments, or chemical substances that impart colour or formed colours added to food, drink, pharmaceuticals, etc. (Newsome et al., 2014). As the quality of food is an aesthetical appeal issue thus colourants have been employed to improve food organoleptic characteristics for thousands of years. A wide variety of food colourants have been employed either from natural or synthetic sources; among them, azo dyes are very common. Up to now, more than 3000 azo dyes have been reported in the world, and in the food industry, among all the synthetic colourants, azo dyes constitute about 65% of commercial market volume (Li et al., 2018). Food products are artificially coloured for making attractive food mixtures to lure consumers because they not only attract but enhance appetite. Natural food colourants have limited application in food industries because of many disadvantages including high cost, poor colouring ability, ease of discolouration and many more. On the other hand, synthetic food colourants are brightly coloured and stable and thus are extensively employed over natural food colourants. Different countries and regions have strict legislations for types, application scopes, and standard limits of the synthetic food colourants that are approved for human consumption. Because of the few varieties and relatively high price of the approved natural and synthetic food colourants, industrial food colours with the features of strong colouring ability and low price have been illegally added in food products by some of the vile food manufacturers, and their uses are continuously reported by the researchers (Dixit et al., 2013; Ashok et al., 2017; Li et al., 2018).

The use of colourants in food products is subjected to a wide range of toxicity tests including acute, sub-chronic, and chronic toxicity, carcinogenicity, mutagenicity, teratogenicity, etc. (Mittal et al., 2007). To evaluate the potential toxicity of food colourants, preclinical studies were conducted by the investigators to determine the no observed adverse effect level (NOAEL) (Amchova et al., 2015). For this reason, food safety authorities summarize all possible data which concern from the health point of view and suggests whether it is permeable or not. The toxicological data on food colourants must be confirmed in six animal species and three out of them must be mammalian which are close to the human body physiology. Pre-clinical data from animal studies confirm the NOAEL. NOAEL quantity is then divided by safety factor, which is usually 100 to determine the acceptable daily intake (ADI) (Bhatt et al., 2018). Such precautions and care cannot eliminate the risk of possible adverse reactions to a particular substance, especially concerning vulnerable populations or hypersensitive individuals. Concern rises regarding human health effects especially in children when the consumption of visibly alluring food products such as cotton candy, soft drinks, flavoured chips, cereals (corn flakes, muesli, etc.), cake mixes, soups, sauces, some rice, ice cream, chewing gum, jam, jelly, and curry is higher in the younger population.

A study reported by Goldenring et al. (1982) proved that biotransformed products (amines) of synthetic food colourants can cross the blood-brain barrier and alter brain physiology. The free radical production resulting from exposed chemicals generally increased chemical and enzymatic oxidation of dopamine and this has been evident from postmortem and clinical investigations. Aromatic amines can enhance the production of reactive oxygen species through interfering in antioxidant defense mechanism which is well established by several studies and generally showed an increase in lipid peroxidation and decline in the activity of superoxide dismutase (SOD) and catalase (CAT) in the brain tissue (Bhatt et al., 2018). Several preclinical, as well as some clinical studies, reported that azo food colourants can cause neurotoxicity and altered the behaviour of humans and animals (McCann et al., 2007; Amchova et al., 2015).

It has long been suggested that synthetic colours and other additives may affect children's behaviour (Overmeyer and Taylor, 1999). In this regard, a study involving 3 and 8–9-year-old children were conducted, which has the greatest impact on the existing legislation and published in 2007, in which six synthetic food colours: Sunset Yellow, Azorubine, Tartrazine, Ponceau 4R, Quinoline Yellow, and Allura Red were used to evaluate the effects on changes in the behaviour of children. The results showed that the intake of these colours harmed children's activity and attention (McCann et al., 2007). Since then, several countries; Irish study (Connolly et al., 2010) focused on the exposure of food colourants to the children, India (Dixit et al., 2011), Kuwait (Husain et al., 2006), and the US (Doell et al., 2016) began to explore more to determine the effects of food colours on humans with special emphasis on whether it can cause attention deficit hyperactivity disorder (ADHD).

To construct systematic knowledge on the neurotoxicity of azo food colourants, it is obvious to gather which described the neurotoxicity of azo food colourants. So, recent literature with a brief description on the neurotoxicity of azo food colourants; neurobehavioural (ADHD, learning and memory and motor), oxidative stress, neurochemical changes, effects on apoptotic and other proteins, and histopathological changes in the brain has been extensively reviewed. Keeping in view the exposure pattern of azo food colourants, the present book chapter is aimed to provide brief and systematic knowledge about the neurotoxicity induced by the azo food colourants in exposed individuals.

Behavioural Abnormalities

Cognition is the ultimate function of the brain and is broadly defined as the sum of mental processes of acquiring knowledge through problem-solving, memory, perception, and planning (Robbins, 2011). It is estimated that at present more than 47 million people have cognitive impairments and this percentage is continuously rising and could be tripled by 2050, shockingly, 60% of 47 million people are from low to middle-income countries (WHO, 2015). Cognitive impairments occur across a range of processes such as attention, learning, and memory and executive functions such as planning and problem-solving. It can lead to a decrease in quality of life, a loss of independence which impacts individuals, their families, the healthcare system, and society as a whole. Furthermore, cognitive impairment can also occur in 'healthy' individuals under certain conditions such as sleep deprivation, malnutrition and through other sporadic factors like environmental pollutants, food additives especially artificial food colourants, etc. which affects both function and economy (Colten and Altevogt, 2006). Azo food colourants induced neurobehavioural alteration in clinical and pre-clinical studies has been summarized in Table 1.

Attention Deficiency Hyperactivity Disorder (ADHD) and Other Motor Dysfunctions

For survival, organisms evolve to detect changes in the environment. Due to limited neural resources, all the information cannot enter conscious awareness. ADHD is one of the most common behavioural disorders in children, affecting 3–7% of school-aged children (Pashler, 2016). As defined by the Diagnostic and Statistical Manual of Mental Disorders of the American Psychiatric Association, the essential features of ADHD include a pervasive pattern of hyperactivity-impulsivity and/or inattention, which is observed before the age of 7 years and occurs for a minimum of 6 months. Hyperactivity and/or in-attention must occur in two or more settings (e.g., school and home), and there must be evidence of developmentally inappropriate social, academic, or occupational functioning. In day-to-day life, these features translate into children facing difficulties on focusing tasks, sitting still, listening to and following instructions, organizing tasks, and processing the information as quickly and accurately as others. Children with ADHD may also be impatient, often interrupting others' conversations, blurting out inappropriate comments, and displaying their emotions without restraint.

Table 1. Azo food colourants induced neurobehavioral alterations

Name of azo food colourants	Type of study	Neurotoxicity	Reference
Tartrazine	Clinical trial	Irritability, restlessness, and sleep disturbance	Rowe and Rowe, 1994
Sunset yellow, tartrazine, carmoisine, and ponceau 4R	Clinical trial	ADHD	Bateman et al., 2004
Tartrazine	Pre-clinical	Hyperactivity and Learning and memory	Tanaka, 2006
Sunset yellow, carmoisine, tartrazine, allura red and ponceau	Clinical trial	ADHD	McCann et al., 2007
Tartrazine	Pre-clinical	Learning and memory	Gao et al., 2011
Brilliant blue	Pre-clinical	Hyperactivity	Tanaka et al., 2012
Ponceau 4R, allura red AC, sunset yellow, tartrazin, amaranth and azorubin	Pre-clinical	Learning and memory	Doguc et al., 2012
Allura red, tartrazine and sunset yellow	Pre-clinical	Hyperactivity	Erickson et al., 2014
Allura red	Pre-clinical	Learning and memory	Noorafshan et al., 2018
Tartrazine	Pre-clinical	Locomotors activity	Albasher et al., 2020
Metanil yellow, malachite green and sudan III	Pre-clinical	Locomotors activity (Balance and coordination)	Pronit et al., 2021

ADHD; attention-deficit hyperactivity disorder.

Artificial food colourants have long been suggested to adversely affect behaviours, especially overactive, impulsive, and inattentive behaviour (i.e., hyperactivity). Ben Feingold made his initial claims of the negative effect of synthetic food colourants on childhood behaviour about 45 years ago and hypothesized that hyperactivity might be a child's adverse reaction to food additives including synthetic colours. Since then different kinds of synthetic food colourants including azo food colours have been studied separately or in mixture form for behavioural changes in experimental studies (Arnold et al.,

2012). In this regard, Tanaka and his group give extensive scientific experimental contributions for pre-clinical analysis of behavioural alterations on exposure of azo food colourants (Tanaka et al., 2012).

Initially, Feingold suggested that the food additive (including artificial food colours) might be the reason for hyperactivity in the children; even his study results conclude the hypothesis. During 1970 to 1980s his claims had potential in the scientific community and most of the studies supported Feingold's original findings. However, the observation made by the clinician, parents, teachers, and researchers were expected the finding. To eliminate the expectation of Feingold's study, a diet replacement study in which two diets with one contained food colour additive were applied. Subjects responded positively when the diet with food additive was given after the control diet. Several researchers have also been engaged in the review of past literature with artificial food colours a meta-analysis and suggested ADHD in their conclusion (Kanarek, 2011). A report of two European studies in which diets that eliminated artificial food colour suggested a significant increase in hyperactive behaviour with the artificial food colourants (Schab and Trinh, 2004; Bateman et al., 2004). McCann reported that when azo food colourants were administered to the children (3 years and 8/9 years) for a 1-week, a small significant composite of overactivity in all children has been noticed (McCann et al., 2007).

To evaluate the effect of prenatally exposed tartrazine on motor behaviour of mice offspring, Albasher et al. (2020) treated mice during pregnancy and 15 days after birth. The result of the study suggests that prenatally exposed mice offspring showed increased locomotion in the locomotor activity test. There were no such studies that suggested the effects of azo food colourant on gender but Tanaka, (2006) reported that male offspring showed a higher significant effect on the exploratory behaviour in juvenile male mice in a dose-related manner. Recently Biswas et al. (2021) reported that when rats were treated with azo food colourants, the stride length, forelimb and hindlimb overlap, and maximum difference between shortest and highest stride length has been significantly changed and concluded that the treatment group faced balance and coordination problems.

Learning and Memory Deficits

Memory is defined as the process by which experienced-based information is encoded, stored, and retrieved. It is one of the most fundamental mental processes that support all of our daily functions beyond simple reflexes and stereotyped behaviours; it is largely what makes each human unique. It is one of the most important forms of higher cognitive processing required for survival. Loss of memory (dementia) not only has distressing personal consequences, but it is also a major social and financial burden on society. It is a key symptom in numerous neurodegenerative diseases (Hippius and Neundorfer, 2003). These diseases are typically associated with the dysfunction of certain neuromodulatory systems; the cholinergic system in AD and the dopaminergic system in schizophrenia and PD (Nagpure and Bian, 2015). Short-term memory is the capacity to temporarily hold a limited amount of information in a very accessible state (Lukács et al., 2016). Spatial memory refers to the storage and retrieval of information about one's surroundings and its spatial orientation, vital for navigation (Olton, 2018). As an animal navigates its environment and landmark cues are used to construct a coherent spatial representation of the environment in memory.

When rats are treated with a high dose of Allura red, results of novel objects recognition and eight-arm radial maze test for memory suggests impairment (Noorafshan et al., 2018). Gao et al. (2011) suggested that tartrazine (permitted food colourants) when treated to the rat and mice, there have been an increase in the escape latency and decrease in the retention latency in the Morris water maze test, indicated that deficits in learning and memory. When a mixture of Erythrosine, Ponceau 4R, Allura Red AC, Sunset Yellow FCF, Tartrazine, Amaranth, Brilliant Blue, Azorubin, and Indigotin before and during the gestation, special and working memory have been reduced in the offspring (Doguc et al., 2012). N-methyl- D-aspartate receptors (NMDARs) and nicotinic acetylcholine receptors (nACHRs) have important for learning and memory and Ceyham et al. (2013) established that the neurogenesis of nAChR β2 and nAChR α4 receptor have been altered in rat's offspring on exposure in gestation.

Oxidative Stress-Induced Toxicity

Inhibition of Complex I or III of the mitochondrial electron transport chain causes an increase in the release of electrons from the transport chain into the mitochondrial matrix which then reacts with oxygen to form reactive oxygen species (ROS) such as ·O2-, hydroxyl radicals (·OH) and nitrogen species (NO·). Leakage occurs by blockage of electron movement along the chain to the next acceptor molecule (Lambert and Brand, 2004). The formed ROS can act as signaling molecules by causing lipid peroxidation or can promote excitotoxicity and both can lead to modification of proteins and eventual cell death of a cell. There has been evidence explained this mechanism of cell death in azo food colourants induced toxicity and can alter biochemical markers (MDA, GSH, SOD, and catalase), mitochondrial complex enzyme (I and II), and neurotransmitters (gamma-aminobutyric acid, dopamine, and serotonin) in the brain. Azo food colourants induce oxidative stress through free radical production, disrupts the mitochondrial respiratory chain, and ATP production via depletion of intracellular NAD+ stores (Bhatt et al., 2018; Mohamed et al., 2015; Biswas et al., 2021; Albasher et al., 2020).

The most common mechanisms of protein damage caused by ROS are oxidations in which carbonylation and nitration of proteins take place. ROS can readily oxidize amino acids of various cellular proteins to form carboxyl groups which can disrupt the physiological function of the affected protein and lead to cytotoxic protein aggregates followed by activation of cell death pathways and impairment of neuroprotective pathways (Esrefoglu, 2009). An increase in these carbonyl groups has been reported in the basal ganglia and prefrontal cortex suggesting a role in the disease. Peroxynitrite is formed by the reaction of ROS with nitric oxide and can nitrate tyrosine residues on proteins (Reiter et al., 2000), damaging them and leading to cell death. ROS (Smit and Anderson, 1992) can also oxidize sulphydryl groups on glutathione, leading to depletion of antioxidant defenses and other thiol-containing co-factors, disrupting various cellular processes and structures. The detailed mechanism of oxidative stress-induced neurotoxicity is represented in Figure 1.

Lipid peroxidation is another main type of cellular damage caused by ROS when reacting with the hydrogen of the lipid and leading to the formation of lipid radicals. This radical can form further lipid radical via an intermediary reaction with hydrogen leading to a chain reaction. Cell membrane phospholipids are susceptible to this damage due to their polyunsaturated nature and leading to damage of both cell and organelle membranes. There has been a strong link between increased lipid peroxidation in the brain with increased levels of malondialdehyde which represents the cause of neuronal cell death and suggests a role for it in the mechanisms of neuronal death (Bhatt et al., 2018; Biswas et al., 2021).

This oxidative damage could be exacerbated in azo food colourants toxicity by the discovery of reduced antioxidant defenses in rats. The mainline of evidence relates to reduced GSH, which is selectively decreased in the brain regions (Rafati et al., 2017), leading to a decline in cellular capability to inactivate H_2O_2 and peroxynitrite. There have been consistent reports of changes in the levels of most of the other major antioxidant systems; SOD and CAT (Bhatt et al., 2018; Biswas et al., 2021). Iron is an integral component of all respiratory chain complexes and its uptake by the brain is linked with mitochondrial energy demand. It has been reported that iron involved in the production and propagation of oxidative stress and increased iron levels in the brain have long been associated with neurodegenerative pathology. Although, increases might be the effect of normal pathological clearance of iron during cell death which occurs in neurodegenerative disease. ROS can increase the release of reactive ferrous iron from this ferritin so leading to the creation of more ROS via the Fenton reaction and increasing oxidative stress and cell damage. The evidence in which abnormal iron homeostasis in several neurodegenerative diseases is clear but the role of iron either as an initiator or a consequence of pathology remains to be elucidated (Gille and Reichmann, 2011).

Neurochemicals Changes

Neurotransmitters play unique trophic roles in the development of the brain. Accordingly, many drugs and environmental toxicants that promote or interfere with neurotransmitters at production levels induce neurodevelopmental abnormalities by disrupting the intensity of neurotrophic activity (Xing and Huttner, 2020). Acetylcholine (Ach), gamma-aminobutyric acid (GABA), dopamine (DA), glutamate, and serotonin (5HT) are considered to be the most important neurotransmitters and control the behaviour. ACh and glutamate control cognitive functions; GABA is an inhibitory neurotransmitter that slows down the actions of the neurons; DA appears to control the voluntary movements of the body and 5HT controls the mood, emotion, and anxiety of the subjects (Lovheim, 2012). Mohamed et al. (2015) reported that treatment of tartrazine reduced the levels of neurotransmitters (GABA, DA, and 5HT) in the brain tissue. When a sub-lethal concentration of basic red (an azo dye) is treated to the zebrafish in their early-life stages, the activity of acetylcholinesterase enzyme (AChE) has been downed compared to control and affects locomotors activity (Abe et al., 2018). When rats treated with metanill yellow, malachite green, sudan III, and their mixture to the activity of monoamine oxidase B (MAO-B), (responsible for the metabolic fate of dopamine in dopaminergic neurons) significantly changed compared to the control. Also AChE activity has been found higher in the treatment group compared to the control (Biswas et al., 2021).

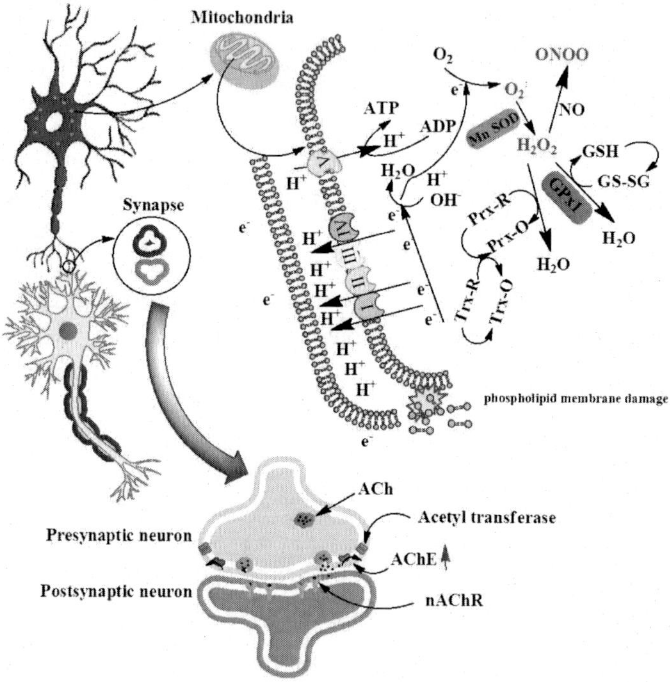

Figure 1. Schematic representation of azo food colourants induced free radical generation, oxidative damage and cholinergic neurotransmitters alteration. Azo food colourants enhance the free radical production, leaked electron reacts to oxygen to form superoxide radical ($O2^{\cdot-}$) which then converted to hydrogen peroxide (H_2O_2) by the SOD. H_2O_2 then react with ferrous iron (Fe^{2+}) to form hydroxide radical ($^{\cdot}OH$). These ROS damages the mDNA, protein and lipid membrane, increasing further mitochondrial ROS production in a vicious cycle. Mitochondria contain several antioxidants enzymes that safely scavenge these ROS. Manganese superoxide dismutase, dismutase $O_2^{\cdot-}$ into oxygen and H_2O_2 which is then oxidized into the water by mitochondrial glutathione peroxidase (GPx1), leading to the oxidation of reduced GSH into glutathione disulfide (GSSG), GSSG then reduced back into GSH by GSH reductase. Within the mitochondrial respiratory chain, electrons are sequentially transferred to different polypeptide complexes (numbered from I to IV) embedded within the inner membrane. The final transfer of the electrons to oxygen takes place at the level of complex IV which oxidizes cytochrome c. The flow of electrons within the MRC is coupled with the extrusion of protons (H^+) from the mitochondrial matrix to the intermembrane space, which creates the mitochondrial transmembrane potential. When energy is needed (i.e., when ATP levels are low), these protons re-enter the matrix through complex V, thus liberating energy that is used to phosphorylate ADP into ATP. In cholinergic nerve synapses, Acetylcholinesterase enzyme (AChE) activity is enhanced thus post synapse Acetylcholine neurotransmitter (Ach) is shorted for cognitive signals transmission. nAChR; nicotinic acetylcholine receptor.

Apoptosis and Other Molecular Markers

Immunohistochemical staining of the cerebral cortex of rat's brain shows higher anti-ssDNA antibody (an apoptotic cell marker) in the tartrazine treated group compared to the control (Mohamed et al., 2015). Another study in which tartrazine has been treated to rats for investigation of histopathological, immunohistochemical on proliferating cell nuclear antigen (PCNA), and glial fibrillar acidic protein (GFAP) showed intense expression of GFAP PCNA in the nuclei of the acinar in the cerebellum in the treated group compared to the control (El-sakhawy et al., 2019). N-methyl-D-aspartate receptors (NMDARs) and nicotinic acetylcholine receptors (nACHRs) are effective in the learning and memory generating process. To investigate the effects of a mixture of food colourants; Erythrosine, Ponceau 4R, Allura Red AC, Sunset Yellow, Tartrazine, Amaranth, Brilliant Blue, Azorubin, and Indigotin on the expression of NMDARs and nACHERs in fat rats showed higher expressions of NR2B and nAChR $\beta 2$ whereas expression of nAChR $\alpha 4$ has been significantly decreased in the male experimental group compared to control. In the case of females, the mixture caused a decrease in NR2B expression compared to the control group (Ceyhan et al., 2013). On the neurological safety aspect, an *In vitro* pathological study on mouse NB2a neuroblastoma cells line revealed that neurite inhibited with the involvement of N-methyl-D-aspartate (NMDA) receptors (Lau et al., 2006).

Histopathological Changes

The high dose of azo food colourants can induce a reduction in the volume of the medial prefrontal cortex and its subdivision, number of neurons and glial cells, and enhanced the mushroom and thin spines per dendrite length with numerous apoptotic cells (Rafati et al., 2017; Mohamed et al., 2015). It has been observed that when rats administered azo food colourants, numerous pyknotic nuclei in the cerebral cortex and neuronal damage in the cerebrum, medulla, and degenerative Purkinje cells with morphologic abnormalities in cellular architecture (El-sakhawy et al., 2019; Albasher et al., 2020; Biswas et al., 2021). Prenatal exposure of azo food colourants to the offspring results in characteristic motor activity and anxiety-like behavioural changes which indicates that development and ageing can be vulnerable with those periods in the life of offspring (Erickson et al., 2014). Allura red, tartrazine, sunset yellow, amaranth are permitted food colourants but the preclinical study on neural progenitor cell toxicity express quite a contrast results. Neural progenitor cells; a biomarker for developmental stage, and neurogenesis indicative of the function of the adult central nervous system (CNS) have been changed on exposure to azo food colourants. Exposure to these food colourants in mouse developing CNS model shows reduced neural progenitor cells and viability and decreased in newly generated cells in the hippocampus of adult mice indicates the potential adverse effects on hippocampal neurogenesis (Park et al., 2009). When Allura red was treated to the rat, it induced damages to the medial prefrontal cortex structure, loss of the cortex volume, and dendrites (Noorafshan et al., 2018). Recently, Biswas et al. (2021) reported that when rats were treated with Metanil Yellow, Malachite Green, Sudan III and the mixture of these three non-permitted food colourants, the cellular architecture of Purkinje cells; responsible for motor coordination and balance have been deformed in the shape, shrunken and degenerated.

Conclusion

The use of food colourants has been a long practice in food products and industrial revaluation makes a huge impact for use of artificial food colours. Although most azo dyes are carcinogenic, other toxicities cannot be neglected. With the gradual accumulation of scientific data on toxicities, the scientific community forces to put these colourants under prohibition and regulation guidelines. Behavioural impairments especially ADHD due to the consumption of food colourants come to light more than 40 years but the South Hamptons studies put a great impact on the scientific community. In recent years, it has been observed that data on neurotoxicity research in food colourants induced toxicity continuously growing and strengthen to rethink the use of food colourants. The patterns of neurotoxicity reported in most of the literature are around oxidative stress, but with this, it is hard to deduce a broad knowledge that very specifically concludes on neurotoxicity. Hence, there is a strong mechanism-based study need to be carried out associates the findings of behavioural abnormalities with mitochondrial dysfunction and oxidative stress, and their biogenesis, neurotrophic factors, receptors and neurotransmitters involved in behavioural alterations and their neurogenesis.

Acknowledgments

The authors are thankful to Dr. Harisingh Gour Vishwavidyalaya (A Central University), Sagar, (MP), India for providing the opportunity to work and their support and interest. Mr. Pronit Biswas is thankful to the University Grant Commission (UGC), New Delhi, India for providing a research fellowship.

Consent for Publication

Not Applicable.

Conflict of Interest

The author confirms that this chapter's contents have no conflict of interest.

References

Abe, Flavia R., Amadeu MVM Soares, Danielle P. de Oliveira, and Carlos Gravato. "Toxicity of dyes to zebrafish at the biochemical level: cellular energy allocation and neurotoxicity." *Environmental pollution* 235 (2018): 255-262. https://doi.org/10.1016/j.envpol.2017.12.020.

Albasher, Gadah, Najla Maashi, Saleh Alfarraj, Rafa Almeer, Tarfa Albrahim, Fatimah Alotibi, May Bin-Jumah, and Ayman M. Mahmoud. "Perinatal exposure to tartrazine triggers oxidative stress and neurobehavioural alterations in mice offspring." *Antioxidants* 9, no. 1 (2020): 53. https://doi.org/10.3390/antiox901 0053.

Amchova, Petra, Hana Kotolova, and Jana Ruda-Kucerova. "Health safety issues of synthetic food colourants." *Regulatory toxicology and pharmacology* 73, no. 3 (2015): 914-922. http://dx.doi.org/10.1016/j.yrtph.2015.09.026.

Arnold, L. Eugene, Nicholas Lofthouse, and Elizabeth Hurt. "Artificial food colours and attention-deficit/hyperactivity symptoms: conclusions to dye for." *Neurotherapeutics* 9, no. 3 (2012): 599-609. https://doi.org/10.1007/s13311-012-0133-x.

Ashok, Vipin, Nitasha Agrawal, Josep Esteve-Romero, Devasish Bose, and Neeti Prakash Dubey. "Detection of Methyl Orange in Saffron and Other Edibles Using Direct Injection Micellar Liquid Chromatography." *Food Analytical Methods* 10, no. 1 (2017): 269-276. https://doi.org/10.1007/s12161-016-0578-3.

Aston-Jones, Gary, and Jonathan D. Cohen. "An integrative theory of locus coeruleus-norepinephrine function: adaptive gain and optimal performance." *Annu. Rev.*

Neurosci. 28 (2005): 403-450. https://doi.org/10.1146/annurev.neuro.28.061604.135709.

Bateman, Belinda, John O. Warner, E. Hutchinson, Taraneh Dean, P. Rowlandson, C. Gant, Jane Grundy, C. Fitzgerald, and J. Stevenson. "The effects of a double blind, placebo controlled, artificial food colourings and benzoate preservative challenge on hyperactivity in a general population sample of preschoolchildren." *Archives of disease in childhood* 89, no. 6 (2004): 506-511. http://dx.doi.org/10.1136/adc.2003.031435.

Bäumler, Wolfgang. "Absorption, distribution, metabolism and excretion of tattoo colourants and ingredients in mouse and man: the known and the unknown." *Curr Probl Dermatol* 48 (2015): 176-184. https://doi.org/10.1159/000369222.

Bhatt, Diksha, Krati Vyas, Shakuntala Singh, P. J. John, and Inderpal Soni. "Tartrazine induced neurobiochemical alterations in rat brainsub-regions." *Food and chemical toxicology* 113 (2018): 322-327. https://doi.org/10.1016/j.fct.2018. 02.011.

Biswas, Pronit, Whidul Hasan, Juli Jain, Rajesh Kumar Kori, Devasish Bose and Rajesh Singh Yadav. "Non-Permitted Food Colourants Induced Neurotoxicity in Cerebellum of Rat Brain." *Drug and Chemical Toxicology*. 2021. (Accepted Manuscript).

Bresciani, Guilherme, Ivana Beatrice Mânica da Cruz, and Javier González-Gallego. "Manganese superoxide dismutase and oxidative stress modulation." *Advances in clinical chemistry* 68 (2015): 87-130. https://doi.org/10.1016/bs.acc. 2014.11.001.

Ceyhan, Betul Mermi, Fatih Gultekin, Duygu Kumbul Doguc, and Esin Kulac. "Effects of maternally exposed colouring food additives on receptor expressions related to learning and memory in rats." *Food and chemical toxicology* 56 (2013): 145-148. https://doi.org/10.1016/j.fct.2013.02.016.

Colten, Harvey R., and Bruce M. Altevogt. "Sleep physiology." In *Sleep disorders and sleep deprivation: An unmet public health problem*. National Academies Press (US), 2006. Bookshelf ID: NBK19956.

Connolly, A., A. Hearty, Anne Nugent, Aideen Mckevitt, Elaine Boylan, Albert Flynn, and M. J. Gibney. "Pattern of intake of food additives associated with hyperactivity in Irish children and teenagers." *Food Additives and Contaminants* 27, no. 4 (2010): 447-456. https://doi.org/10.1080/19440040903470718.

Dixit, Sumita, S. K. Purshottam, S. K. Khanna, and Mukul Das. "Usage pattern of synthetic food colours in different states of India and exposure assessment through commodities preferentially consumed by children." *Food Additives & Contaminants: Part A*28, no. 8 (2011): 996-1005. https://doi.org/10.1080/194400 49.2011.580011.

Dixit, Sumita, Subhash K. Khanna, and Mukul Das. "All India survey for analyses of colours in sweets and savories: exposure risk in Indian population." *Journal of food science* 78, no. 4 (2013): T642-T647. https://doi.org/10.1111/1750-3841.120 68.

Doell, Diana L., Daniel E. Folmer, Hyoung S. Lee, Kyla M. Butts, and Susan E. Carberry. "Exposure estimate for FD&C colour additives for the US population." *Food Additives & Contaminants: Part A*33, no. 5 (2016): 782-797. https://doi.org/10.1080/ 19440049.2016.1179536.

Doguc, Duygu Kumbul, Betul Mermi Ceyhan, Mustafa Ozturk, and Fatih Gultekin. "Effects of maternally exposed colouring food additives on cognitive performance in rats." *Toxicology and industrial health* 29, no. 7 (2013): 616-623. https://doi.org/10.1177/0748233712436638.

Duffus, John H., Monica Nordberg, and Douglas M. Templeton. "Glossary of terms used in toxicology, (IUPAC Recommendations 2007)." *Pure and Applied Chemistry* 79, no. 7 (2007): 1153-1344. https://doi.org/10.1351/pac200779071153.

El-Sakhawy, Mohamed A., Dina W. Mohamed, and Yasmine H. Ahmed. "Histological and immunohistochemical evaluation of the effect of tartrazine on the cerebellum, submandibular glands, and kidneys of adult male albino rats." *Environmental Science and Pollution Research* 26, no. 10 (2019): 9574-9584. https://doi.org/10.1007/s11356-019-04399-5.

Erickson, Zachary T., Erin A. Falkenberg, and Gerlinde AS Metz. "Lifespan psychomotor behaviour profiles of multigenerational prenatal stress and artificial food dyeeffects in rats." *PloS One* 9, no. 6 (2014): e92132. https://doi.org/10.1371/ journal.pone.0092132.

Esrefoglu, Mukaddes. "Oxidative stress and benefits of antioxidant agents in acute and chronichepatitis." *Hepatitis monthly* 12, no. 3 (2012): 160. https://dx.doi.org/10.5812%2Fhepatmon.837.

Gao, Yonglin, Chunmei Li, Jingyu Shen, Huaxian Yin, Xiulin An, and Haizhu Jin. "Effect of food azo dye tartrazine on learning and memory functions in mice and rats, and the possible mechanisms involved." *Journal of food science* 76, no. 6 (2011): T125-T129. https://doi.org/10.1111/j.1750-3841.2011.02267.x.

Gille, Gabriele, and Heinz Reichmann. "Iron-dependent functions of mitochondria—relation to neurodegeneration." *Journal of neural transmission* 118, no. 3 (2011): 349-359. https://doi.org/10.1007/s00702-010-0503-7.

Goldenring, J. R., D. K. Batter, and B. A. Shaywitz. "Sulfanilic acid: behavioural change related to azo food dyes in developing rats." *Neurobehavioural toxicology and teratology* 4, no. 1 (1982): 43-49. PMID: 6803178.

Hippius, Hanns, and Gabriele Neundörfer. "The discovery of Alzheimer's disease." *Dialogues in clinical neuroscience* 5, no. 1 (2003): 101. https://dx.doi.org/10.31887%2FDCNS.2003.5.1%2Fhhippius.

Husain, A., W. Sawaya, A. Al-Omair, S. Al-Zenki, H. Al-Amiri, N. Ahmed, and M. Al-Sinan. "Estimates of dietary exposure of children to artificial food colours in Kuwait." *Food additives and contaminants* 23, no. 3 (2006): 245-251. https://doi.org/10.1080/02652030500429125.

Kanarek, Robin B. "Artificial food dyes and attention deficit hyperactivity disorder." *Nutrition reviews* 69, no. 7 (2011): 385-391. https://doi.org/10.1111/j.1753-4887.2011.00385.x.

Lambert, Adrian J., and Martin D. Brand. "Inhibitors of the quinone-binding site allow rapid superoxide production from mitochondrial NADH: ubiquinone-oxidoreductase (complex I)." *Journal of Biological Chemistry* 279, no. 38 (2004): 39414-39420. https://doi.org/10.1074/jbc.M406576200.

Lau, Karen, W. Graham McLean, Dominic P. Williams, and C. Vyvyan Howard. "Synergistic interactions between commonly used food additives in a developmental neurotoxicity test." *Toxicological sciences* 90, no. 1 (2006): 178-187. https://doi.org/10.1093/toxsci/kfj073.

Li, Yongxin, Yi Yang, Shuo Yin, Chen Zhou, Dongxia Ren, and Chengjun Sun. "In edible azo dyes and their analytical methods in foodstuffs and beverages." *Journal of AOAC International* 101, no. 5 (2018): 1314-1327. https://doi.org/10. 5740/jaoacint. 18-0048.

Lövheim, Hugo. "A new three-dimensional model for emotions and monoamine neurotransmitters." *Medical hypotheses* 78, no. 2 (2012): 341-348. https://doi.org/ 10.1016/j.mehy.2011.11.016.

Lukács, Ágnes, Enikő Ladányi, Kata Fazekas, and Ferenc Kemény. "Executive functions and the contribution of short-term memory span in children with specific language impairment." *Neuropsychology* 30, no. 3 (2016): 296. https://psycnet.apa. org/doi/ 10.1037/neu0000232.

McCann, Donna, Angelina Barrett, Alison Cooper, Debbie Crumpler, Lindy Dalen, Kate Grimshaw, Elizabeth Kitchin et al. "Food additives and hyperactive behaviour in 3-year-old and 8/9-year-old children in the community: a randomised, double-blinded, placebo-controlled trial." *The lancet* 370, no. 9598 (2007): 1560-1567. https://doi.org/ 10.1016/S0140-6736(07)61306-3.

Mittal, Alok, Lisha Kurup, and Jyoti Mittal. "Freundlich and Langmuir adsorption isotherms and kinetics for the removal of Tartrazine from aqueous solutions using hen feathers." *Journal of hazardous materials* 146, no. 1-2 (2007): 243-248. https://doi.org/10.1016/j.jhazmat.2006.12.012.

Mohamed, Amany Abdel-Rahman, Azza AA Galal, and Yaser HA Elewa. "Comparative protective effects of royal jelly and cod liver oil against neurotoxic impact of tartrazine on male rat pupsbrain." *Acta Histochemica* 117, no. 7 (2015): 649-658. https://doi.org/ 10.1016/j.acthis.2015.07.002.

Mohamed, Samar S., Shereen M. Mahmoud, Rania Abdelrahman Elgawish, and Kawther A. Elhady. "*Sudan III Azo Dye: Oxidative Stress with Possible Geno and Hepatotoxic Effects in Male Rats*." (2016): 1700-1704. https://doi.org/10.21275/ ART20162590.

Nagpure, B. V., and Jin-Song Bian. "Brain, learning, and memory: role of H 2 S in neurodegenerative diseases." *Chemistry, biochemistry and pharmacology of hydrogen sulfide* (2015): 193-215. https://doi.org/10.1007/978-3-319-18144-8_10.

Nakazawa, Kazu, Thomas J. McHugh, Matthew A. Wilson, and Susumu Tonegawa. "NMDA receptors, place cells and hippocampal spatial memory." *Nature Reviews Neuroscience* 5, no. 5 (2004): 361-372. https://doi.org/10.1038/ nrn1385.

Newsome, Andrew G., Catherine A. Culver, and Richard B. Van Breemen. "Nature's palette: the search for natural blue colourants." *Journal of Agricultural and Food Chemistry* 62, no. 28 (2014): 6498-6511. https://doi.org/10.1021/jf5014 19q.

Noorafshan, Ali, Maedeh Hashemi, Saied Karbalay-Doust, and Fatemeh Karimi. "High dose Allura Red, rather than the ADI dose, induces structural and behavioural changes in the medial prefrontal cortex of rats and taurine can protect it." *Acta histochemica* 120, no. 6 (2018): 586-594. https://doi.org/10.1016/ j.acthis.2018.07. 004.

Olton, David S. "Characteristics of spatial memory." In *Cognitive processes in animal behaviour*, pp. 341-373. Routledge, 2018.

Overmeyer, Stephen, and Eric Taylor. "Annotation: principles of treatment for hyperkinetic disorder: practice approaches for the UK." *The Journal of Child Psychology and*

Psychiatry and Allied Disciplines 40, no. 8 (1999): 1147-1157. https://doi.org/10.1111/1469-7610.00532.

Park, Mikyung, Hee Ra Park, So Jung Kim, Min-Sun Kim, Kyoung Hye Kong, Hyun Soo Kim, Ein Ji Gong et al. "Risk assessment for the combinational effects of food colour additives: neural progenitor cells and hippocampal neurogenesis." *Journal of Toxicology and Environmental Health, Part* A72, no. 21-22 (2009): 1412-1423. https://doi.org/10.1080/15287390903212816.

Pashler, Harold. *Attention*. Psychology Press, 2016. https://doi.org/10.4324/9781315784762.

Rafati, Ali, Nasrin Nourzei, Saied Karbalay-Doust, and Ali Noorafshan. "Using vitamin E to prevent the impairment in behavioural test, cell loss and dendrite changes in medial prefrontal cortex induced by tartrazine in rats." *Acta histochemica* 119, no. 2 (2017): 172-180. https://doi.org/10.1016/j.acthis.2017.01. 004.

Reiter, Christopher D., Ru-Jeng Teng, and Joseph S. Beckman. "Superoxide reacts with nitric oxide to nitrate tyrosine at physiological pH via peroxynitrite." *Journal of Biological Chemistry* 275, no. 42 (2000): 32460-32466. https://doi.org/10.1074/jbc.M910433199.

Robbins, Trevor W. "Cognition: The ultimate brain function." *Neuropsychopharma-cology* 36, no. 1 (2011): 1-2. https://doi.org/10.1038/npp.2010.171.

Schab, David W., and Nhi-Ha T. Trinh. "Do artificial food colours promote hyperactivity in children with hyperactive syndromes? A meta-analysis of double-blind placebo-controlled trials." *Journal of Developmental & Behavioural Pediatrics* 25, no. 6 (2004): 423-434. https://doi.org/10.1097/00004703-200412 000-00007.

Smit, M. J., and R. Anderson. "Biochemical mechanisms of hydrogen peroxide-and hypochlorous acid-mediated inhibition of human mononuclear leukocyte functions in vitro: protection and reversal by anti-oxidants." *Agents and actions* 36, no. 1 (1992): 58-65. https://doi.org/10.1007/BF01991229.

Tanaka, Toyohito, Osamu Takahashi, Akiko Inomata, Akio Ogata, and Dai Nakae. "Reproductive and neurobehavioural effects of brilliant blue FCF in mice." *Birth Defects Research Part B: Developmental and Reproductive Toxicology* 95, no. 6 (2012): 395-409. https://doi.org/10.1002/bdrb.21029.

Tanaka, Toyohito. "Reproductive and neurobehavioural toxicity study of tartrazine administered to mice in the diet." *Food and Chemical Toxicology* 44, no. 2 (2006): 179-187. https://doi.org/10.1016/j.fct.2005.06.011.

Wang, Szu-Han, and Richard GM Morris. "Hippocampal-neocortical interactions in memory formation, consolidation, and reconsolidation." *Annual review of psychology* 61 (2010):49-79. https://doi.org/10.1146/annurev.psych.093008.100 523.

World Health Organisation. *News: 2015*, WHO 2015. https://www.who.int/news/item/17-03-2015-governments-commit-to-advancements-in-dementia-research-and-care.

Xing, Lei, and Wieland B. Huttner. "Neurotransmitters as modulators of neural progenitor cell proliferation during mammalian neocortex development." *Frontiers in cell and developmental biology* 8 (2020): 391. https://doi.org/10.3389/fcell. 2020.00391.

Chapter 4

Identification of Novel Biomarkers for Neurological Disorders: A Computational Approach

Sunil Kumar Gupta[1,*] and Sarita Singh[2]

[1]Department of Pharmacoinformatics,
National Institute of Pharmaceutical Education and Research, Hyderabad, Telangana, India

[2]Bioinformatics Centre, Biotech Park, Sector-G, Jankipuram, Lucknow, Uttar Pradesh, India

Abstract

Neurological disorders are the significant arena among the health care researchers worldwide, as illnesses like Parkinson's, Alzheimer's, Dementia, Schizophrenia, Motor neuron disease and Huntington's disease, people have to live out with the disability throughout their life. Neurological disorders are multifactorial diseases such as genetic, environmental chemicals like pesticides and metals, etc. Biomarkers can be useful on early detection and invigilation of the disease progression as well as sensitivity to environmental chemicals and reaction to therapeutic interventions. Various biomarkers for neurological disorders have been identified in laboratory and translated with the clinical studies. Computational and bioinformatics approaches have also been used by some of them. Up to now, no perfect biomarker is available, which can help in early detection, follow up on treatment and identifying the vulnerable populations. Therefore, an effort has been made to review study the advancements in computational approaches for finding the novel biomarkers and their validation. Computational methods have

* Corresponding Author's Emails: skgupta.res@gmail.com; sunil.gupta1@niperhyd.ac.in.

In: New Perspectives in Neuroscience
Editors: Prachi Srivastava, Neha Srivastava and Prekshi Garg
ISBN: 978-1-68507-754-9

potential to make available rapid and accurate approach to get novel biomarkers.

Introduction

Neurological disorders is the second leading cause of death after heart disease with 9 million deaths and with 276 million disability-adjusted life-years (DALYs), it is the leading cause of disability, worldwide (GBD project, 2020). WHO reported that neurological disorders affect more than 450 million people globally from 1990 to 2016. In India 30 million people suffers from various forms of neurological diseases and the average prevalence rate is as high as 2,394 per 100,000 of the population. In human it includes a wide range of disorders like Alzheimer disease (AD), Parkinson disease (PD), Dementia, Motor neuron disease (MND), Schizophrenia and Huntington's disease (HD), etc. Most of them shares common symptom & neuro-pathological conditions. Therefore, it becomes quite challenging to diagnose a particular disorder (Ward et al. 2010). Hence, it is necessary to understand the molecular mechanism and pathological symptoms of disease to foresee the same. A WHO report estimated that in 2015 neurological disorders contributed to 95 million disability-adjusted life-years (DALY) which was projected to reach to 103 million in 2030 worldwide.

Biomarkers are helpful in the early diagnostics and follow-up of disease advancement and also vulnerability to environmental chemicals and response to therapeutic interventions. The term "biomarker," was making known in 1960s regarding biochemical and metabolites irregularities allied with several ailments. According to Naylor's definition "A characteristic that is objectively measured and evaluated as an indicator of normal biological processes, pathogenic processes, or pharmacologic responses to a therapeutic intervention" is biomarker (Naylor 2003). The 'Bence Jones' a protein in urine was identified as cancer biomarker in 1847, which was the first biomarker tested in lab (Jain 2010). In simple language biomarker is a measurable biological entity that associates with a physiological, pathological or clinical opinion. It could be genes, gene products, hormones, enzymes, specific cell, etc. Alterations in biological structures and organ's functions could also be a biomarker. Besides, some biomarkers with therapeutic effect are also accessible (Ransohoff 2003; Riesterer 2007; Kim et al. 2008). Novel biomarkers are required to define the stages of disease progression to comprehend the disease pathology in detail. For disease progression sensitivity, specificity and inconsistency of biomarkers should be described appropriately and also validated as risk predictor (Ward et al. 1996).

With the recent advances the computational approaches assimilate multi-omics data to understand new underlying disease mechanisms that leads to biomarker discovery and their clinical validation. The application of computational biology in neurological disorder helps to collect information regarding structure and function of control against diseased brain by obligingomics data like genomics, proteomics, metabolomics and transcriptomics. This will provide deeper insight mechanism of the complex feature of CNS that affected by various factors. It is well known that nervous system is a complex sophisticated system, also making the study of biomarkers of neurological diseases complicated. Hence computational methods may rapid up the search of potential biomarkers. Therefore, the current study focused on computational approaches in novel biomarker discovery associated with neurological disorder based on knowledge driven approaches.

Computational Approaches for Biomarker Identification

Rapid advancements in molecular and information technologies have jointly generated significant data associated with molecular biology of any disease. The key goal of bioinformatics is to better understand of biological processes (Raza 2010). It plays a vital role to point out the clinical dares in early diagnosis, prognosis and effective therapies in neurological diseases. Computational tools/software and databases could be helpful to explore the molecular machines of any disease and identify the authentic as well as specific biomarkers.

It can be able researchers and clinicians to response the important queries based on the details of individual patient like characteristics of the disease, laboratory testing results, multiomics information, etc. Computational methods have an important role in drug discovery via correlation study of the individual findings such as experimental design, study implementation and biochemical analysis. It also helps in translational research for transforming data into medical practice and inspires the development of new drugs and biomarkers through providing critical tools. Advancement of cost-effective, offensive diagnostic tests after their validation will aided both the medical practitioner and patients using bioinformatics approach (Suh et al. 2013). Only few of the neurological biomarkers identified through computational approaches have been validated in clinical trials (Table 1).

Table 1. Biomarkers identified using computational approaches

Disease	Biomarker	Reference
Parkinson's Disease	HLF, E2F1 and STAT4 NUCKS1	Diao et al. 2012 Sarita et al. 2019
Alzheimer's Disease	SEC22B, RAB10, FLT1 genes SNPs i.e., rs7530069, rs113464261, rs114506298, rs73504429, rs7929589, rs76306710, rs66813 BDNF and WWTR1 *Choline acetyltransferase *Urokinase-type plasminogen activator receptor	Zhao et al. 2016, Sherif et al. 2015, Greco et al. 2012 Yu et al. 2021
Huntington's disease (HD)	FNDC3A, BCLAF1 and ALCAM	Chakraborty et al. 2021
Neurodegeneration	ULK1	Garg et al. 2020

*Biomarkers clinically validated

Numerous databases and computational methods are available for novel biomarker identification which utilize the multi-omics data and identified the appropriate marker for disease progression. The flow chart of the study is given in Figure 1.

A. Multi-Omics and Neuroimaging Databases

Various public repositories with huge data related to neurological disorders are available (Table 2). PubMed, PubMed central and Medline have research articles published by researchers. Sequential data like DNA/gene, RNA/mRNA, Protein, whole genome, ESTs, etc. are available at NCBI and UniProt. Similarly GO database have gene ontology data and Gene Omnibus and Array Express contains gene expression data. KEGG database systematically integrates genomic and chemical information while PANTHER provides a structured representation of protein function in the context of biological reaction networks. Alzheimer's disease Neuroimaging Initiative (ADNI) and Biomarkers for Alzheimer's and Parkinson's disease database (BIOMARKAPD) databases are being used, to test the magnetic resonance imaging (MRI), positron emission tomography (PET), and other biological markers which helps in prediction of AD and PD in early stages. Besides, GOBIOM, the world's largest Biomarker database contains over 74,000 biomarkers for 18 different disorders, has been developed by GVK

Biosciences, Hyderabad, India. These databases are significant resources for retrieving anticipated datasets for biomarker identification.

Table 2. Multi-omics and neuroimaging databases for neurological biomarker discovery

Name of Database	Source Link
National Centre for Biotechnology Information (NCBI)	www.ncbi.nlm.nih.gov
UniProt	www.uniprot.org
PubMed/ PubMed central	www.ncbi.nlm.nih.gov/pubmed
Medline	www.medline.com
Gene Ontology (GO)	www.geneontology.org
Gene Expression Omnibus (GEO)	www.ncbi.nlm.nih.gov/geo
WebArrayDB	www.webarraydb.org/webarray
ArrayExpress	www.ebi.ac.uk/arrayexpress/
KEGG (Kyoto Encyclopedia of Genes and Genomes)	www.kegg.jp
PANTHER (Protein Analysis Through Evolutionary Relationships classification system)	www.pantherdb.org
Alzheimer's Disease Neuroimaging Initiative (ADNI)	adni.loni.usc.edu
Biomarkers for Alzheimer's disease and Parkinson's disease (BIOMARKAPD)	www.neurodegenerationresearch.eu
Global Online Biomarker Database (GOBIOM)	gobiomdb.com

B. Literature Mining

A lesser effort has been made to document the information in spite of availability of huge significant information about the disease, technologies developed and prospective drugs for managing the disease, etc. For systematically scrutinize the information warehoused in scientific articles and comprehend their associations with disease progression, the literature mining techniques are progressively advanced. These techniques have enabled the expansion of association networks among numerous biomedical entities such as genes, proteins, drugs and diseases, etc. (Jenssenet al. 2001; Chun et al. 2006; Jensen et al. 2006; Agarwal et al. 2008; Baker et al. 2010; Frijters et al. 2010; Zhu et al. 2010). These computational efforts have been motivated by the vast data generated by high-throughput experiments and its storage in the databases.

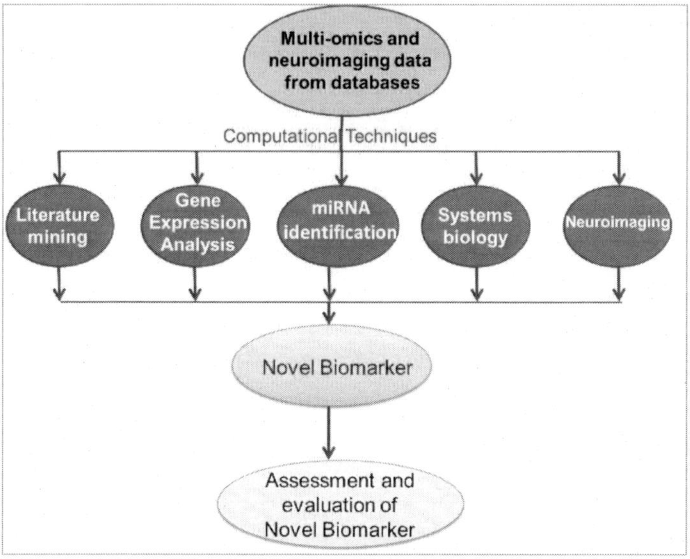

Figure 1. Flow chart for computational methods used for Biomarker identification

The information from literature mining and high-throughput technologies, like microarrays, proteomics, and metabolomics assembled together to support in bio-ontologies construction (Bard et al. 2004; Bodenreider et al. 2006). These ontologies could be assisting in the narration of scientific concepts and their associations like connotation of an existing biomarker/ exposure/drug with a novel diseased condition can also be predictable by passing through ontology (Qu et al. 2009).

Table 3. Tools for literature mining

Text mining tools	Source Link
BioReader	www.cbs.dtu.dk/services/BioReader
Semantic MEDLINE	skr3.nlm.nih.gov/SemMed/index.html
Pubnet	pubnet.gersteinlab.org/
Quertle	www.quertle.com/
Nextbio	www.nextbio.com/
Coremine	www.coremine.com/
LitVar	www.ncbi.nlm.nih.gov/CBBresearch/Lu/Demo/LitVar
Dnorm	www.ncbi.nlm.nih.gov/research/bionlp/Tools/dnorm/
Gnormplus	www.ncbi.nlm.nih.gov/research/bionlp/Tools/gnormplus/
Tmvar	www.ncbi.nlm.nih.gov/research/bionlp/Tools/tmvar/
NegBio	www.github.com/ncbi-nlp/NegBio

Several text mining methods like machine learning or artificial intelligence have also been in use to study the ontologies. The algorithms of the machine learning help to explain the relationships between the features in the data. Consequently, several text mining tools are available to assist in mining appropriate gene or protein data from literature, and these together with manual search have been often found compulsory for functional omics data analyses. Several tools are available for biological data mining as given in Table 3.

C. Gene Expression Analysis

It is a systematic approach with remarkable influence on biological research, pharmacology, and medicine to biological findings. This approach is able to acquire measurable information like the comprehensive transcription profile, to explore the basic biology, disease diagnosis, assist drug advances, alter therapeutics to particular pathologies, and create databases with information related to monitoring procedures of any living individual (Young 2000).

These methods have been supportive in satisfying the gap between DNA sequence and their annotations by dissevering biochemical pathways into intermediary components at genotype and phenotype level. These studies have offers new ways to identify intricate disease genes and biomarkers for disease diagnosis and/or for assessing the efficacy and toxicity of the drug. Application of gene expression analyses in biomarker identification has remarkable role, for disease risk assessment, early stage detection, prognosis, assessing therapeutic response and preventative measures.

Several biomarkers are available for various diseases which have been identified using gene expression analysis methods. Like, PD initiation expression has been identified, using bioinformatics analysis of 1004 differentially co-expressed genes in PD patients compare to controls and pathway enrichment study recommended that protein turn over process were impaired in PD. A regulatory impact factor analysis revealed that some transcription factors like HLF, STAT4 and E2F1 have shown altered expression level in PD patients. Therefore HLF, E2F1 and STAT4 may be used as significant biomarkers after validation (Diao et al. 2012). Also, proteins with tissue-specific expression have also been predicted as cancer serum biomarkers using gene expression analysis (Prassas et al. 2012). Several online tools/software are available for gene expression data analysis. (Table 4)

Table 4. List of some selected tools for gene expression analysis

Gene expression analysis tools	Source Link
BRBArray tool	brb.nci.nih.gov
GEO2R	www.ncbi.nlm.nih.gov/geo/geo2r
CIMminer	discover.nci.nih.gov/cimminer
GEDA	gedas.bizhat.com/gedas.htm
Expression Profiler	www.ebi.ac.uk/expressionprofiler
ArrayQuest	www.proteogenomics.musc.edu/arrayquest
Arraypipe	www.pathogenomics.ca/arraypipe
ASIAN	www.mrc-lmb.cam.ac.uk
CARMAweb	www.mrc-lmb.cam.ac.uk
CARRIE	www.zlab.bu.edu/CARRIE-web
BABELOMICS	www.babelomics.org
DEEP	www.bioinf.med.uni-goettingen.de/services/deep
EagleView	wwsw.niehs.nih.gov

D. miRNA Analysis

MicroRNA (miRNA), is a small nucleotide sequence that regulate the gene transcription, and aid as indicator for identification and advancement of several diseases. miRNAs have been authenticated in clinical studies of several neurological disorders like, Alzheimer's disease, multiple sclerosis, traumatic brain injuries, Parkinson's disease and CNS tumors as diagnostic markers. miRNAs have numerous features to become a promising candidate biomarkers like stability in body fluids, function in multiple tissues, in pathogenesis, and also the ability to be distinguished initially in the disease progression. Cerebrospinal fluid (CSF) is a favorable source of miRNA in the identification of many neurological disorders due to its cell-free environment, direct contact with the brain and spinal cord and collection process that minimizes tissue damage (Stoicea et al. 2016).

Numerous miRNAs have been recognized as biomarker for diagnosis and treatment of several of diseases using computational approaches. The finding of Cogs well et al., in Alzheimer's disease patient has revealed expression of a different miRNA profiles in the medial frontal gyrus, hippocampus, and cerebellum (Cogswell et al., 2008). miRNA-AD/PD connotations in domestic animals i.e., cow, pig, horse and chicken using computational methods have been reported which offers researcher to generate AD/PD models using domestic animal for further studies (Wang et al. 2016). 11 miRNAs, have been identified as candidate biomarkers for autism using a knowledge-guided bioinformatics model and validated through literature mining and functional enrichment analyses (Shen et al. 2016).

Several freely accessible virtual databases and tools are available for identification of miRNA for various diseases progression. Some selected miRNA prediction/miRNA target identification tools are mentioned in Table 5. Deregulation in early disease stage, miRNA could be considered a consistent biomarker due to their incidence and stability in body fluids.

E. Systems Biology Approaches

The approaches used to comprehend the mechanism of biological systems to identify specific biomarkers for a certain ailments along with new diseased targets employing computer software, "omics"-based finding tools and progressive concert computational techniques. This method effort to comprehend the interface between several constituents of a specific system via study the relationships within a biological system (Kitano 2002; Hood et al. 2004; Fang et al. 2011; Lucas et al. 2011; Karsenti 2012).

Table 5. List of some selected miRNA analysis databases/tools

miRNA analysis databases/tools	Source Link
MiRBase	www.mirbase.org
MiPred	www.tools4mirs.org
MiRDeep	www.tools4mirs.org/mirdeep
MiRNAFold	www.EvryRNA.ibisc.univ-evry.fr/miRNAFold
mirAnalyzer	www.web.bioinformatics.cicbiogune.es/microRNA
miRanda	www.mirandatools.in
TargetScan	www.targetscan.org
TargetFinder	www.bioit.org.cn/ao/targetfinder
miRWalk	www.zmf.umm.uni-heidelberg.de/apps/zmf/mirwalk2/
miRTarBase	www.miRTarBase.cuhk.edu.cn/.

The progressions in the high-throughput tools and accomplishment of human genome sequencing endorsed gathering and analysis of huge data sets like genomics, proteomics, transcriptomic, etc. (Ideker et al. 2001; Kitano 2002; FDA 2011; Ori et al. 2011). It is assumed that the intricacy of biological systems and datasets acquired by HT techniques could be better understood by using this approach. The development and advancement of new diagnostic tools and therapeutics for several complex diseases, especially neurological disorders, is constrained due to such complexity (Hood et al. 2004; Robeva 2010; Fang et al. 2011; Westerhoff 2011).

In schizophrenia, the lethal effects of GABA that interrupt both the glutaminergic and dopaminergic transmission have been emphasized via application of systems biology. Besides in Bipolar disorder, systems biology revealed the association of several genes CACNA1C, ANK3, and ITIH3-4 genes via interaction study. Likewise systems biology emphasized a connection between synaptic perturbations and cognitive impairments in autism (Vattikuti et al. 2010).

To model biological systems, the systems biology approach utilizes publically available or innovative computational tools and resources (Alawieh et al. 2012). It empowers a superior aptitude to recognize the inter-dependencies between the pathways of disease, and the intricacy of the systems. This approach may possibly be valuable tool for determining specific biomarkers for a particular disease. Some specific system biology tools are listed below (Table 6).

Table 6. List of some popular data resources and tools for systems biology

System biology tools	Source Link
Cytoscape	www.cytoscape.org
Reactome	www.reactome.org
Network Analyst	www.networkanalyst.ca
MiRNet	www.mirnet.ca
GeneMANIA	www.genemania.org
Kyoto Encyclopedia of Genes and Genome (KEGG)	www.kegg.jp
Protein Analysis Through Evolutionary Relationships classification system(PANTHER)	www.pantherdb.org
Search Tool for the Retrieval of Interacting Genes Proteins (STRING)	www.string.embl.de
Pathway Analyser	sourceforge.net/ projects/ pathwayanalyser
WikiPathways	wikipathways.org
Ingenuity Pathways Analysis (IPA)	www.ingenuity.com
Institute of Medicinal Molecular Design (KeyMolnet)	www.immd.co.jp

F. Neuroimaging

Neuroimaging data has been analyzed using *in-silico* algorithms, also for identification of genetic biomarkers. For example, the polymorphisms in the genes associated with AD exploiting different Bayesian network structure learning algorithms for detecting the causal ADSNPs and gene-SNP interactions was studied and new SNP biomarkers were perceived to be considerably allied with AD (Sherif et al. 2015). Several neuroimaging software/tools are available to study the structure and function of the normal vs. diseased brain (Table 7).

Table 7. List of preferred neuroimaging tools

Neuroimaging Tools	Source Link
3DSlicer	www.slicer.org
Analysis of Functional NeuroImages (AFNI)	www.afni.nimh.nih.gov
FMRIB Software Library (FSL)	www.fsl.fmrib.ox.ac.uk/fsl/fslwiki/FSL
Multi-Image Analysis GUI (Mango)	www.ric.uthscsa.edu/mango
CONN (functional connectivity toolbox)	www.web.conn-toolbox.org
LONI Pipeline	www.pipeline.loni.usc.edu

Computational methods employing above listed databases, investigation tools and techniques offer an exceptional prospect to evaluate markers distinctly for prognostic, diagnostic and response predictive values for neurological disease, rapidly. Platform based techniques that used entail several years to complete, but now it will take a few weeks or months by a trained bio informatician. Now sets of markers that might characterize regulatory pathways or other molecular functions can be assessed rather single biomarker. The compound data sets also make available a prospect optimization of marker in a data set and liberated validation in several others. Besides the efficacy and accuracy of the biomarker is also important for the clinical viewpoint. It helps us to know whether the new biomarker is safe for clinical use or not. The key parameter for evaluation includes area under the curve (AUC) of receiver operating characteristics (ROC) curve, sensitivity and specificity. There are several computational tools are available for the assessment of newly identified biomarker based on the above said statistical parameters like Stata 8 (www.stata.com), Decision Curve Analysis (www.mskcc.org) and Risk Prediction Package (www.research.fhcrc.org), etc. At present in India, several research laboratories are focusing on computational biomarkers identification for numerous cancer types like Institute of Bioinformatics, Bangalore, National Institute of Immunology, New Delhi and many others.

Limitations

Each procedure or methods have their own limitations. A significant constraint to computational method is that consistency of the outcomes produced by computational analysis using publicly accessible data is reliant on the reliability of the source data. It is also challenging to authenticate the precision of clinical explanations. Inconsistencies in measurements can be vital and logical variances in the investigative procedures affect the assessments among datasets. Hence, a biomarker revealed completely through computational methods is implausible to acquire widespread clinical approval. If there is difference between high throughput platform and anticipated clinical methods then authentication of the new analyses alongside the inventive outcomes is needed. Likewise, however miRNA analysis gain advantages, presently investigative tools are so far expensive as a clinically feasible for analytical process and require standardization (Stoicea et al. 2016). Mining of literature is also a significant aspect of the data analysis workflow and several literature mining tools are available for the assistance of appropriate data mining from literature manually, while none is incorporated with omics system in a way that data extracted using computational methods can be used for functional exploration, directly (Hu et al. 2011). However, different types of biomarkers like genetic, epigenetic, biochemical, environmental which used as primitive, prognostics, diagnostics markers, etc. have been recognized using computational methods but a drug responders and non-responders biomarker to identify computationally, is still a dare. Consequently it is another constraint of computational technique and it can only be done in-vivo at present.

The biomarker has presumed a great significance and will be more by researchers and clinicians both in academia and industries, in future. The application of computational methods for identification of biomarker, are assured to advances the understanding of disease pathway and factors affecting them. Specificity and validation of the biomarkers, in future may also be predicted using computational approaches which will diminish the dependencies on wet lab.

Conclusion

Fast progression in computational algorithms and high throughput data is a good prospect to identify the novel cost effective biomarkers, rapidly. These could be further employed for probable validation of clinical data. This chapter describes that computational technology, with limitations, have advantages above other approaches. Keeping in view the complexity of nervous system, biomarker prediction particularly for neurological diseases, these computational methods gains noteworthy advantage. Several new algorithms based on biological data extracted from available databases with improved biomarker selection measures should be developed to get novel biomarkers with high specificity and sensitivity.

References

Agarwal, P. and Searls, D.B. (2008). Literature mining in support of drug discovery. *Briefings in Bioinformatics*, *9* (6), 479-492.

Alawieh, A., Zaraket, F.A., Li, J., Mondello, S., Nokkari, A., Razafsha, M., Fadlallah, B., Boustany, R. and Kobeissy, F.H. (2012). Systems biology, bioinformatics, and biomarkers in neuropsychiatry. *Frontiers in Psychiatry*, *6* (187), 1-16.

Baker, N.C. and Hemminger, B.M. (2010). Mining connections between chemicals, proteins, and diseases extracted from Medline annotations. *Journal of Biomedical Informatics*, *43* (4), 510-519.

Bard, J.B. and Rhee, S.Y. (2004). Ontologies in biology: design, applications and future challenges. *Nature Review of Genetics*, *5* (3), 213-222.

Bodenreider, O. and Stevens, R. (2006). Bio-ontologies: current trends and future directions. *Briefings in Bioinformatics*, *7*(3), 256-274.

Chakraborty, S. (2021). Identification of Blood Based Bio-Marker for Huntington's disease using *in-silico* gene expression analysis. *bioRxiv* https://doi.org/10.1101/ 2021.03.26.437248.

Cogswell, J.P., Ward, J., Taylor, I.A., Waters, M., Shi, Y. and Cannon, B. (2008). Identification of miRNA changes in Alzheimer's disease brain and CSF yields putative biomarkers and insights into disease pathways. *Journal of Alzheimer's Disease*, *14*, 27–41.

Diao, H., Li, X., Hu, S. and Liu, Y. (2012). Gene Expression Profiling Combined with Bioinformatics Analysis Identify Biomarkers for Parkinson Disease. *PLoS One*., *7*(12), e52319.

Fang, F.C. and Casadevall, A. (2011). Reductionist and holistic science. *Infection and Immunity*, *79*, 1401-1404.

Food and Drug Administration, H.H.S. (2011). International conference on harmonisation; guidance on E16 biomarkers related to drug or biotechnology product development: context, structure, and format of qualification submissions; availability. *Federal Register*, *76*, 49773-49774.

Frijters, R., Van, V.M. and Smeets, R. (2010). Literature mining for the discovery of hidden connections between drugs, genes and diseases. *PLoS Computational Biology*, *6* (9), 1-11.e1000943.

Garg, P., Srivastava N., Seth, P.K., Srivastava, P. (2021). *In silico* study of ULK1 gene as a susceptible biomarker for neurodegeneration. *Annals of Neurosciences*. (In press)

Greco, I., Day, N., Riddoch, C. J., Reed, J., Soininen, H., Oszewska, I.K., Tsolaki, M., Vellas, B., Spenger, C., Mecocci, P., Wahlund, L.O., Simmons, A., Barnes, J. and Lovestone, S.S. (2012). Alzheimer's disease biomarker discovery using *in silico* literature mining and clinical validation. *Journal of Translational Medicine.*, *10*, 217.

Hood, L. and Perlmutter, R.M. (2004). The impact of systems approaches on biological problems in drug discovery. *Nature Biotechnology*, *22*, 1215-1217.

Hu, Z., Huang, H., Wu, C.H., Jung, M., Dritschilo, A., Riegel, A.T. and Wellstein, A. (2011). Omics-based molecular target and biomarker identification. *Methods in Molecular Biology*, *719*, 547-571.

Ideker, T., Galitski, T. and Hood, L. (2001). A new approach to decoding life: systems biology. *Annual Review of Genomics and Human Genetics*, *2*, 343-372.

Jain, K.K. (2010). *The Handbook of Biomarker*. Boston, Springer publication.

Jensen, L.J., Saric, J. and Bork, P. (2006). Literature mining for the biologist: from information retrieval to biological discovery. *Nature Reviews Genetics*, *7*(2), 119-129.

Jenssen, T.K., Laegreid, A. and Komorowski, J. (2001). A literature network of human genes for high-throughput analysis of gene expression. *Nature Genetics*, *28*(1), 21-28.

Karsenti, E. (2012). Towards an "oceans systems biology". *Molecular Systems Biology*, *8* (575), 1-2.

Kim, Y.S, Maruvada, P. and Milner, J.A. (2008). Metabolomics in biomarker discovery: future uses for cancer prevention. *Future Oncology*, *4*, 93–102.

Kitano, H. (2002). Systems biology: a brief overview. *Science*, *295*, 1662-1664.

Lucas, M., Laplaze, L. and Bennett, M. J. (2011). Plant systems biology: network matters. *Plant*, *Cell & Environment*, *34*, 535–553.

Naylor, S. (2003). Biomarkers: current perspectives and future prospects. *Expert Review of Molecular Diagnostics*, *3*, 525–529.

Ori, A., Wilkinson, M.C. and Fernig, D.G. (2011). A systems biology approach for the investigation of the heparin/heparan sulfate interactome. *Journal of Biological Chemistry*, *286:* 19892-19904.

Prassas, I., Chrystoja, C.C., Makawita, S. and Eleftherios, P. (2012). Bioinformatics identification of proteins with tissue-specific expression for biomarker discovery. *BMC Medicine*, *10* (39), 1-13.

Qu, X.A., Gudivada, R.C. and Jegga, A.G. (2009). Inferring novel disease indications for known drugs by semantically linking drug action and disease mechanism relationships. *BMC Bioinformatics*, *10* (Suppl 5), S4.

Ransohoff, D.F. (2003). Cancer. Developing molecular biomarkers for cancer. *Science*, *299*, 1679–1680.

Raza, K. (2010). Application of Data Mining in Bioinformatics. *Indian Journal of Computer Science and Engineering*, *1* (2), 114-118.

Riesterer, O., Milas, L. and Ang, K.K. (2007). Use of molecular biomarkers for predicting the response to radiotherapy with or without chemotherapy. *Journal of Clinical Oncology*, *25*, 4075–4083.

Robeva, R. (2010). Systems biology - old concepts, new science, new challenges. *Frontiers in Psychiatry*., *1*(1), 1-2.

Shen, L., Lin, Y., Sun, Z., Yuan, X., Chen, L. and Shen, B. (2016). Knowledge-guided bioinformatics model for identifying autism spectrum disorder diagnostic microRNA biomarkers. *Scientific Reports*, *6*, 39663: 1-9.

Sherif, F.F., Zayed, N. and Fakhr, M. (2015). Discovering alzheimer genetic biomarkers using Bayesian networks. *Advances in Bioinformatics*, *639367*, 1-8.

Singh, S., Seth, P.K. (2019). Functional association between NUCKS1 gene and Parkinson disease: A potential susceptibility biomarker. *Bioinformation*, 15(8):548-556.

Stoicea, N., Du, A., Lakis, D.C., Tipton, C., Arias-Morales, C.E. and Bergese, S.D. (2016). The miRNA journey from theory to practice as a CNS biomarker. *Frontiers in Genetics*, *7* (11), 1-8.

Suh, K.S., Sarojini, S., Youssif, M., Nalley, K., Milinovikj, N., Elloumi, F., Russell, S., Pecora, A., Schecter, E. and Goy, A. (2013). Tissue banking, bioinformatics, and electronic medical records: the front-end requirements for personalized medicine. *Journal of Oncology*, *368751*, 1-12.

Vattikuti, S. and Chow, C.C. (2010). A computational model for cerebral cortical dysfunction in autism spectrum disorders. *Biological Psychiatry*, *67*, 672–678.

Wang, H.A., Lin, Z.L., Yu, X.F., Bao, Y., Cui, X. and Kim, N. (2016). Computational prediction of Alzheimer's and Parkinson's disease microRNAs in domestic animals. *Asian Australasian Journal of Animal Sciences.*, *29* (6), 782-792.

Ward, J.B. Jr. and Henderson, R.E. (1996). Identification of needs in biomarker research. *Environmental Health Perspectives*, *104*, Supplement 5.

Ward, M., Schofield, E.L. (2010). Biomarkers for brain disorders. *Therapy, 7*(4):321-336.

Westerhoff, H. V. (2011). Systems biology left and right. *Methods in Enzymology*, *500*, 3-11.

Young, R.A. (2000). Biomedical discovery with DNA arrays. *Cell*, *102*, 9-15.

Yu, W., Yu, W., Yang, Y., Lü, Y. (2021). Alzheimer's disease, diagnosis biomarkers, hubgenes, integrative analysis, aging. *Frontiers in Aging Neuroscience*, 13: 1663-4365.

Zhao, Y., Tan, W., Sheng, W. and Li, X. (2016). Identification of biomarkers associated with Alzheimer's disease by bioinformatics analysis. *American Journal of Alzheimer's Disease and Other Dementias*, *31*(2), 163-168.

Zhu, Q., Lajiness, M.S. and Ding, Y. (2010). WENDI: a tool for finding non-obvious relationships between compounds and biological properties, genes, diseases and scholarly publications. *Journal of Chemoinformatics*, *2* (6), 1-9.

Chapter 5

miRNA and Mammalian Circadian Clock: A Crosstalk

Anshul Tiwari[1,*] and Prachi Srivastava[2]
[1]Channing Division of Network Medicine, Brigham and Women's Hospital, Harvard Medical School, Boston, Massachusetts, USA
[2]Amity Institute of Biotechnology, Amity University
Uttar Predesh, Lucknow, India

Abstract

Circadian clocks are endogenous oscillators that regulate behavior and physiology across a 24-hour cycle in order to accomplish time-dependent balance with the external environment. Transcription–translation feedback loops, along with post-transcriptional and post-translational modification, are being used to generate the systems. Current findings reveal that additional non-coding RNA-based processes are necessary to keep the clock functioning efficiently. MicroRNAs are a critically essential element in the regulation of circadian rhythm and many other physiological activities. Circadian inequality not affects our sleeping cycle and periodic physiological activity, but it also correlates with the development of conditions such as insomnia and neurodegenerative diseases. MicroRNA dysfunction is rapidly being documented as a source of sporadic neurodegenerative disorders via unregulated genes involved in neurodegenerative disease pathogenesis, and involvement of some genes are also found in the development of inherited neuro-degenerative disorders. Here, we explore possible ways of unlocking microRNAs' usefulness as effectors of circadian physiology and

* Corresponding Author's Email: anshulmbi@gmail.com.

In: New Perspectives in Neuroscience
Editors: Prachi Srivastava, Neha Srivastava and Prekshi Garg
ISBN: 978-1-68507-754-9

pathology based on recent research indicating a critical role for microRNAs in neurodegenerative disease and clock physiology.

Introduction

Physiology and behavior in mammals and other animals are regulated by an innate molecular clock that is synchronized with the 24-hour solar day (Lowrey and Takahashi 2004). The ability to accommodate to the rotation of our planet by relying on the sun's cycles is an ancient characteristic (Tosches et al. 2014). This phenomenon illustrates why the proper circadian clock's operation is extremely important for physiological activities in any of our body's tissues, and why disruptions in the latter can significantly contribute to chronic multifactorial diseases. Circadian rhythm has far-reaching implications that go beyond neuronal activity, hormonal release and feeding behavior (Pivovarova et al. 2016). This pace-making system has an effect on every cell in our body, so each tissue or organ maintains its circadian rhythm despite metabolic or environmental stressors that occur throughout our lives (West and Bechtold 2015). The highest hierarchical unit, which is located on the bottom of the anterior hypothalamus and represents a tiny region named the suprachiasmatic nucleus (SCN), commands these tissues to reset their internal clock. It responds to environmental and physiological changes in order to keep and synchronize the clocks all over our body (Eckel-Mahan et al. 2013). All mammals, including humans, have a circadian clock that regulates their sleeping and feeding patterns (Preussner and Heyd 2016).

Non-coding RNAs (ncRNAs) are a popular topic in science right now. Several non-coding RNAs are extremely valuable in living systems and use different ways to compensate for their incapability to be translated into proteins. MicroRNAs (miRs) are a type of non-coding RNA that acts as a post-transcriptional regulator. miRs have a role in the control of a broad range of factors important to the body's biological processes (Cora' et al. 2017). It is evidential through current findings that miRs regulate gene expression circadian rhythms and inversely (Cheng et al. 2007). The circadian clock's molecular mechanism is tightly controlled by post-transcriptional and post-translational regulation, which is centered on a disciplined transcription and translation response loop.

Clock gene (s) govern the circadian clock, further expression, and oscillation of most of these genes are also regulated. There are numerous physiological functions stay governed by circadian regulation, which is achieved by the recurring of gene expression regulation. Experimental animals missing the clock gene (s) are alive and reproducible, indicating that a malfunction of the circadian clock is not lethal to living species (Tsang et al. 2017). The circadian clock system's failure has been connected to a number of health problems. Neurological issues for example sleep disturbances and neurodegenerative disorder might result from a central nervous system breakdown. Sleep disruption is a typical initial indication of disease of the nervous system; as a result, it could play a role in the beginning and development of the disease. Furthermore, improperly expressed miRNAs in the blood, body fluids, and/or some tissues are frequently seen in individuals with sleep disturbances as well as patients with illnesses of the nervous system (Piletič and Kunej 2016). These findings suggest that miRNAs, through modifying the genes expression associated with or contributing to disorders, might perhaps be used as biomarkers for disease pathogenesis as well as effective therapies.

Circadian Rhythm and Neurodegenerative Diseases: Is There a Link?

The slow degradation of the nervous system's structure and function is defined by neurodegenerative illnesses such as amyotrophic lateral sclerosis (ALS), Parkinson's disease (PD), and Alzheimer's disease (AD). No neurodegenerative disease is currently curable; the present therapies merely address the symptoms or reduce the disease's development. The global increase in life expectancy and the subsequent growth in the older population increased the percent ratio of neurodegenerative diseases and illnesses as compared to others. These diseases primarily affect people in their later years of life. Circadian irregularities have long been thought to be a consequence of neurodegeneration. According to new studies, circadian disturbance might be a factor in the neurodegenerative process (Kondratova and Kondratov 2012). The circadian clock may have a straighter part in the initiation of neurodegenerative disorders, according to many research. (Videnovic and Zee 2015).

There are different factors that contribute to the beginning and development of neurodegenerative disorders, oxidative stress is one of them (Niedzielska et al. 2015). Most of the genes that govern the antioxidant system, interestingly, have a circadian rhythm (Kinoshita, Aoyama, and Nakaki 2018). BMAL1-deficient mice also reveal greater levels of reactive oxygen species (ROS) and age quicker, indicating the involvement of the circadian clock in ROS control (Kondratov 2006). Imbalance of reductant and oxidant (Redox) situations are classified as oxidative stress in which the formation of reactive oxygen species outpaces the antioxidant systems' capacity to control it (Henchcliffe and Beal 2008). miRs are one of the most essential RNA-processing factors, and they regulate post-transcriptional processes (Bartel 2009). Patients with neurodegenerative disorders have abnormal miRNA expression in their brains, cerebrospinal fluid, and blood (Renoux and Todd 2012).

Amyotrophic Lateral Sclerosis (ALS)

It is a chronically progressive disease distinguished by particular motor neuron degradation in the spinal cord and motor cortex that typically leads to death within 3-5 years of onset (Gordon 2013). ALS patients, the cortisol cycle is disrupted; specifically, cortisol values in the evening are much greater in ALS patients than in healthy people. (Patacchioli et al. 2003).

Abundant genes have been revealed to contain mutations that might be hereditary factors that might cause ALS, according to a study. Some of them comprise mutations in the TAR DNA-binding protein 43 (TDP-43), Cu/Zn superoxide dismutase 1 (SOD1), chromosome 9 open reading frame 72 (C9orf72) and fused in sarcoma/translated in liposarcoma (FUS) (Taylor, Brown, and Cleveland 2016). Circadian variations in SOD1 expression and activity are drastically reduced in Per1/Per2 double-knockout (DKO) mice (Jang et al. 2011). TDP-43 also controls the circadian clock by maintaining CRY proteins (Hirano et al. 2016). The new FUS modulator for circadian gene expression has recently been identified to have positive control on REV-ERB (Jiang et al. 2018). Circulating miRs may have a function in the ALS pathology's linkage of central and peripheral organs since ALS appears to affect not just neurons in the CNS but also peripheral muscle tissues. The most promising circulating miRNAs that are affected in ALS patients are miR-206 and miR-133a/b. In ALS patients, expression of both of these miRs are significantly noticed in myocytes and are raised in muscle and brain (Ricci, Marzocchi, and Battistini 2018).

Other miRs have been proven to target particular genes associated to ALS development, such as miR-142 and miR-132 (Ricci, Marzocchi, and Battistini 2018). In sporadic ALS patients, miR-142 levels are elevated in the spinal cord (Figueroa-Romero et al. 2016). MiR-142 has been associated to TDP-43 and

C9orf72 and regulates the expression of Nrf2, a transcription factor that affects the expression of antioxidant-response genes (Matamala et al. 2018, Nguyen, Nioi, and Pickett 2009). Both miRs, miR-133a and miR-133b, are very much expressed in ALS patients and contributed to muscle proliferation, repair, and regeneration (Figueroa-Romero et al. 2016, Raheja et al. 2018, Tasca et al. 2016). Based on the major differences discovered between a clock mutant and wild type fly, it has been proven that miR-133, which is highly conserved, leads to core circadian gene expression (Xia et al. 2019). ALS patients have been shown to have higher levels of miR-206, and it is thought to contribute to the reinnervation process (Ma et al. 2015). MiR-206 also has a substantial influence on the mammalian circadian clock's dynamic mechanism, affecting both the amplitude and frequency of gene expression changes (Zhou et al. 2011). These findings imply that ALS-causing genes and circadian genes and miRs are closely connected.

Parkinson's Disease

Following Alzheimer's disease, it is the most prevalent neurodegenerative disorder, as well as being clinically distinct by resting tremor, stiffness, akinesia, and postural instability (Hayes 2019). A progressive, late-onset mobility disability is caused by dopaminergic neurodegeneration in the substantia nigra (SN). Eosinophilic neuronal inclusions containing both -synuclein and ubiquitin are pathogenic indicators of Parkinson's disease (Ascherio and Schwarzschild 2016). Diurnal variations in dopamine and certain of its metabolites have been documented in several studies. Dopamine content fluctuations could be linked to cycles in dopamine producing enzymes and transporters, whose activity alter throughout time (Sleipness, Sorg, and Jansen 2007). The circadian clock can govern rhythmic dopaminergic activity, which could in turn regulate the clock's activity (Mendoza and Challet 2014, Sleipness, Sorg, and Jansen 2007). Dopamine may potentially play a function in the circadian retinal input regulation (Witkovsky 2004). In many recent studies, several miRs were discovered to be dysregulated in the entire blood, serum, and CSF of patients with PD. According to a recent study, people with Parkinson's disease had lower levels of miR-30c expression (Roser et al. 2018). Patients with narcolepsy exhibit greater levels of miR-30c, and in juvenile narcoleptics, alteration in MiR-30c expression in response to lack of sleep have been discovered (Holm et al. 2014, Weigend et al. 2018). Despite the fact that the precise targets of miR-30c have yet to be discovered, an analytical method indicated a number of target genes implicated in neuronal autophagy, mitophagy, and dopaminergic cell death regulation (Vallelunga et al. 2019). Furthermore, circadian PER proteins are predicted to be miR-30c target genes (Figueredo et al. 2013), albeit the exact mechanisms by which miR-30c influences PD pathogenesis and circadian rhythm remain unknown.

Furthermore, the members of the miR-29 family are particularly remarkable in this regard, since together miR-29a and miR-29c transcripts are down-regulated in Parkinson's disease (Terrinoni et al. 2018). Interestingly, blood miR-29a is upregulated in levodopa-treated PD patients (Serafin et al. 2015), and Overexpression of miR-29c in the SN of Parkinson's disease mice decreased dopaminergic neuron loss and accumulation of synuclein, according to research (Wang et al. 2019). The miR-29 family's targets also include PER proteins, albeit the miR-29 family's rhythmicity has yet to be discovered (Chen, D'Alessandro, and Lee 2013, Figueredo et al. 2013). miR-29 family members have been hypothesized as crucial participants in neurodegeneration and clock gene dysregulation because their expression is changed in Alzheimer's patients.

Patients with Parkinson's disease are compared to healthy control groups, they also have substantially lower amounts of miR-221. miR-221 protects against Parkinson's disease by targeting an apoptosis-related gene and is regulated by DJ-1, whose impairment variation are connected to recessively inherited PD (Li et al. 2018). Furthermore, the expression of miR-221 in salivary has been discovered to oscillate throughout the day, suggesting that circadian dysregulation of anti-inflammatory actions via miRNAs may play a role in PD pathogenesis (Hicks et al. 2018). These findings point to a link between PD etiology, oxidative stress, and miRNA dysregulation in the causation of Parkinson's disease.

Alzheimer's Disease

Alzheimer's disease (AD) is an irreparable age-related neurodegenerative disease distinguished by progressive dementia that manifests later in life or in middle age. Pathological indicators in the brain include amyloid (A) plaques and neurofibrillary tangles generated by tau protein that has been inappropriately phosphorylated (Stakos et al. 2020). Insomnia, nighttime arousal, numerous wakefulness and awake too early morning, and drowsiness naps are all prevalent Alzheimer's disease symptoms. In people with Alzheimer's disease, obstructive sleep apnea is also frequent (Brzecka et al.

2018). These problems are also present in patients with moderate cognitive impairment, implying that sleep difficulties may be basic signs before to the diagnosis of Alzheimer's disease. Due to a straightening of the melatonin rhythm, there are minor changes between daytime and nighttime bouts of activity and sleep in extreme situations. Cortisol release patterns have also been seen to change.

There have been reports of aberrant BMAL1 methylation and transcription in Alzheimer's disease patients' brains, resulting in altered BMAL1 expression and neuronal circadian rhythms, which lead to sleep and behavior disorders (Cronin et al. 2017). Furthermore, Bmal1 controlled the activity of the APOE gene in an Alzheimer's disease animal model, and Bmal1 omission resulted in a loss of oscillations in the hippocampus, subsequent in large elevations in amyloid plaque burden (Kress et al. 2018). Aβ, surprisingly, exhibits a diurnal rhythm, with a raised amount during waking and a lower level during sleep (Huang et al. 2012). Aβ circadian pattern decline with age and amyloid accumulation have also been documented.

It's worth mentioning that mutual miRs are linked to the gene expression involved in circadian rhythm, sleep disorders, and Alzheimer's disease pathogenesis, implying a strong relationship. miR-219 expression has been reported to be higher in the Alzheimer's patients' brains, and miR-219 is recognized to have a contribution in the suppression of Tau phosphorylation via targeting GSK-3β (Arnes et al. 2019). Through the CLOCK and BMAL1 complex, this miRNA has been shown to modulate the circadian clock (Cheng et al. 2007). In Alzheimer's disease, miR-132 is substantially downregulated in neurons (El Fatimy et al. 2018). GSK-3 and Tau mRNA are targets of miR-132, which may be triggered by photic entrainment cues through a MAPK/CREB-dependent pathway. miR-146a, on another side, is upregulated in numerous brain areas in Alzheimer's disease patients (Cheng et al. 2007, Smith et al. 2015, Swarbrick et al. 2019). miR-146a has been connected to insufficient sleep, and its expression has been found to be rhythmic (Davis et al. 2007, Hijmans et al. 2019, Saus et al. 2010, Wang et al. 2014). By altering genes implicated in neuroinflammation and cerebrovascular dysfunction, this miR may also contribute to the development of Alzheimer's disease (Janelidze et al. 2018, Wennstrom and Nielsen 2012). The deregulation of miR-210 in brain tissues, cerebrospinal fluid, and serum has also been linked to the pathogenesis of Alzheimer's disease. Patients with Alzheimer's disease had higher levels of miR-34a in their temporal cortex (Sarkar et al. 2016). miR-34a has been found to have a rhythmic expression pattern in tumor cell lines, and its overexpression causes aberrant expression of the clock genes Per1 and

Per2, as well as genes that have a role in memory development, APP metabolism, and tau phosphorylation states (Han et al. 2016, Hasakova et al. 2019, Sarkar et al. 2019). Despite the fact that miR-125b and miR-29b have been identified as the top-ranking AD biomarkers in numerous clinical investigations, the reason of dysregulation in the blood of AD patients is unclear (Fransquet and Ryan 2018, Liu, Cali, and Lee 2017, Nagaraj et al. 2019). These findings imply that circadian rhythm problems and miRNA dysregulation are significantly linked to AD pathology, etiology, and pathophysiology.

Conclusion and Future Outlook

Circadian changes have recently been linked to the onset of neurodegenerative diseases and may even play a role in disease development, according to new research. As mentioned in the chapter, a growing amount of available data suggests that numerous circadian-related miRNAs are changed in neurodegenerative disorders. Such findings suggest that anomalies in circadian miRNA expression might serve as biomarkers for the development of neurodegenerative diseases in the future. Furthermore, manipulating miRNA expression early throughout the progression of a disease might be utilized to treat neurodegenerative disorders. To discover treatments for neurodegenerative disorder that are now incurable and progressing, further research is required. There is a slew of issues that must be solved before these techniques may be adopted. The inability of RNA constructs (such as antagomirs and sponges) to pass the blood-brain barrier, e.g., is a major roadblock for minimally invasive treatment methods. Additionally, concerns such as antisense administration timing and organ-specific therapeutic targeting will need to be addressed.

References

Arnes, Mercedes, Yoon A. Kim, Jerome Lannes, Maria E. Alaniz, Joshua D. Cho, Brian D. McCabe, and Ismael Santa-Maria. 2019. MiR-219 deficiency in Alzheimer's disease contributes to neurodegeneration and memory dysfunction through post-transcriptional regulation of tau-kinase network. *Cold Spring Harbor Laboratory*.

Ascherio, Alberto, and Michael A. Schwarzschild. 2016. The epidemiology of Parkinson's disease: risk factors and prevention. *The Lancet Neurology 15* (12):1257-1272. doi: 10.1016/s1474-4422 (16)30230-7.

Bartel, David P. 2009. MicroRNAs: Target recognition and regulatory functions. *Cell, 136* (2):215-233. doi: 10.1016/j.cell.2009.01.002.

Brzecka, Anna, Jerzy Leszek, Ghulam Md Ashraf, Maria Ejma, Marco F. Ávila-Rodriguez, Nagendra S. Yarla, Vadim V. Tarasov, Vladimir N. Chubarev, Anna N. Samsonova, George E. Barreto, and Gjumrakch Aliev. 2018. Sleep disorders associated with Alzheimer's disease: a perspective. *Frontiers in Neuroscience, 12*. doi: 10.3389/fnin s.2018.00330.

Chen, Rongmin, Matthew D'Alessandro, and Choogon Lee. 2013. miRNAs are required for generating a time delay critical for the circadian oscillator. *Current Biology, 23* (20):1959-1968. doi: 10.1016/j.cub.2013.08.005.

Cheng, Hai-Ying M., Joseph W. Papp, Olga Varlamova, Heather Dziema, Brandon Russell, John P. Curfman, Takanobu Nakazawa, Kimiko Shimizu, Hitoshi Okamura, Soren Impey, and Karl Obrietan. 2007. microRNA modulation of circadian-clock period and entrainment. *Neuron, 54* (5):813-829. doi: 10.1016/j.neuron.2007.05. 017.

Cora,' Davide, Angela Re, Michele Caselle, and Federico Bussolino. 2017. MicroRNA-mediated regulatory circuits: outlook and perspectives. *Physical Biology, 14* (4):045 001. doi: 10.1088/1478-3975/aa6f21.

Cronin, Peter, Michael J. McCarthy, Andrew S. P. Lim, David P. Salmon, Douglas Galasko, Eliezer Masliah, Philip L. De Jager, David A. Bennett, and Paula Desplats. 2017. Circadian alterations during early stages of Alzheimer's disease are associated with aberrant cycles of DNA methylation in BMAL1. *Alzheimer's & Dementia, 13* (6):689-700. doi: 10.1016/j.jalz.2016.10.003.

Davis, Christopher J., Stewart G. Bohnet, Joseph M. Meyerson, and James M. Krueger. 2007. Sleep loss changes microRNA levels in the brain: A possible mechanism for state-dependent translational regulation. *Neuroscience Letters, 422* (1):68-73. doi: 1 0.1016/j.neulet.2007.06.005.

Eckel-Mahan, K. L., V. R. Patel, S. de Mateo, R. Orozco-Solis, N. J. Ceglia, S. Sahar, S. A. Dilag-Penilla, K. A. Dyar, P. Baldi, and P. Sassone-Corsi.2013. Reprogramming of the circadian clock by nutritional challenge. *Cell, 155* (7):1464-78. doi: 10.1016/j.ce ll.2013.11.034.

El Fatimy, Rachid, Shaomin Li, Zhicheng Chen, Tasnim Mushannen, Sree Gongala, Zhiyun Wei, Darrick T. Balu, Rosalia Rabinovsky, Adam Cantlon, Abdallah Elkhal, Dennis J. Selkoe, Kai C. Sonntag, Dominic M. Walsh, and Anna M. Krichevsky. 2018. MicroRNA-132 provides neuroprotection for tauopathies via multiple signaling pathways. *Acta Neuropathologica, 136* (4):537-555. doi: 10.1007/s00401-018-1880-5.

Figueredo, Diego de Siqueira, Mayara Rodrigues Barbosa, Daniel Leite Góes Gitaí, and Tiago Gomes de Andrade. 2013. Predicted MicroRNAs for mammalian circadian rhythms. *Journal of Biological Rhythms, 28* (2):107-116. doi: 10.1177/0748 730413 476827.

Figueroa-Romero, Claudia, Junguk Hur, J. Simon Lunn, Ximena Paez-Colasante, Diane E. Bender, Raymond Yung, Stacey A. Sakowski, and Eva L. Feldman. 2016. Expression of microRNAs in human post-mortem amyotrophic lateral sclerosis spinal cords provides insight into disease mechanisms. *Molecular and Cellular Neuroscience, 71*:34-45. doi:10.1016/j.mcn.2015.12.008.

Fransquet, Peter D., and Joanne Ryan. 2018. Micro RNA as a potential blood-based epigenetic biomarker for Alzheimer's disease. *Clinical Biochemistry, 58*:5-14. doi: 10.1016/j.clinbiochem.2018.05.020.

Gordon, Paul. 2013. Amyotrophic lateral sclerosis: an update for 2013 clinical features, pathophysiology, management and therapeutic trials. *Aging and Disease, 04* (05):295-310. doi: 10.14336/ad.2013.0400295.

Han, Yuyan, Fanyin Meng, Julie Venter, Nan Wu, Ying Wan, Holly Standeford, Heather Francis, Cynthia Meininger, John Greene, Jerome P. Trzeciakowski, Laurent Ehrlich, Shannon Glaser, and Gianfranco Alpini. 2016. miR-34a-dependent overexpression of Per1 decreases cholangiocarcinoma growth. *Journal of Hepatology, 64* (6):1295-1304. doi: 10.1016/j.jhep.2016.02.024.

Hasakova, Kristina, Richard Reis, Marian Vician, Michal Zeman, and Iveta Herichova. 2019. Expression of miR-34a-5p is up-regulated in human colorectal cancer and correlates with survival and clock gene PER2 expression. *PLOS ONE, 14* (10):e0224396. doi: 10.1371/journal.pone.0224396.

Hayes, Michael T. 2019. Parkinson's disease and parkinsonism. *The American Journal of Medicine, 132* (7):802-807. doi: 10.1016/j.amjmed.2019.03.001.

Henchcliffe, Claire, and M. Flint Beal. 2008. Mitochondrial biology and oxidative stress in Parkinson disease pathogenesis. *Nature Clinical Practice Neurology, 4* (11):600-609. doi: 10.1038/ncpneuro0924.

Hicks, Steven D., Neil Khurana, Jeremy Williams, Cindy Dowd Greene, Richard Uhlig, and Frank A. Middleton. 2018. Diurnal oscillations in human salivary microRNA and microbial transcription: implications for human health and disease. *PLOS ONE, 13* (7):e0198288. doi: 10.1371/journal.pone.0198288.

Hijmans, Jamie G., Ma'ayan Levy, Vinicius Garcia, Grace M. Lincenberg, Kyle J. Diehl, Jared J. Greiner, Brian L. Stauffer, and Christopher A. DeSouza. 2019. Insufficient sleep is associated with a` pro-atherogenic circulating microRNA signature. *Experimental Physiology, 104* (6):975-982. doi: 10.1113/ep087469.

Hirano, Arisa, Tomoki Nakagawa, Hikari Yoshitane, Masaaki Oyama, Hiroko Kozuka-Hata, Darin Lanjakornsiripan, and Yoshitaka Fukada. 2016. USP7 and TDP-43: pleiotropic regulation of cryptochrome protein stability paces the oscillation of the mammalian circadian clock." *PLOS ONE, 11* (4):e0154263. doi: 10.1371/journal.pone.0154263.

Holm, Anja, Claus Heiner Bang-Berthelsen, Stine Knudsen, Birgitte R. Kornum, Signe Modvig, Poul Jennum, and Steen Gammeltoft. 2014. miRNA profiles in plasma from patients with sleep disorders reveal dysregulation of miRNAs in narcolepsy and other central hypersomnias. *Sleep*, 37 (9):1525-1533. doi: 10.5665/sleep.4004.

Huang, Yafei, Rachel Potter, Wendy Sigurdson, Tom Kasten, Rose Connors,John C. Morris, Tammie Benzinger, Mark Mintun, Tim Ashwood, Mats Ferm, Samantha L. Budd, and Randall J. Bateman. 2012. β-amyloid dynamics in human plasma. *Archives of Neurology, 69* (12):1591. doi: 10.1001/archneurol.2012.18107.

Janelidze, Shorena, Niklas Mattsson, Erik Stomrud, Olof Lindberg, Sebastian Palmqvist, Henrik Zetterberg, Kaj Blennow, and Oskar Hansson. 2018. CSF biomarkers of neuroinflammation and cerebrovascular dysfunction in early Alzheimer disease. *Neurology, 91* (9):e867-e877. doi:10.1212/wnl.0000000000006082.

Jang, Yeong-Su, Myung-Han Lee, Sang-Hyuk Lee, and Kiho Bae. 2011.Cu/Zn superoxide dismutase is differentially regulated in period gene-mutant mice. *Biochemical and Biophysical Research Communications, 409* (1):22-27. doi: 10.1016/j.bbrc.2011.04.099.

Jiang, Xin, Tao Zhang, Haifang Wang, Tao Wang, Meiling Qin, Puhua Bao, Ruiqi Wang, Yuwei Liu, Hung-Chun Chang, Jun Yan, and Jin Xu. 2018. Neurodegeneration-associated FUS is a novel regulator of circadian gene expression. *Translational Neurodegeneration, 7* (1). doi: 10.1186/s40035018-0131-y.

Kinoshita, Chisato, Koji Aoyama, and Toshio Nakaki. 2018. Neuroprotection afforded by circadian regulation of intracellular glutathione levels: a key role for miRNAs. *Free Radical Biology and Medicine, 119*:17-33. doi:10.1016/j.freeradbiomed.2017. 11.023.

Kondratov, R. V. 2006. Early aging and age-related pathologies in mice deficient in BMAL1, the core componentof the circadian clock. *Genes & Development, 20* (14):1868-1873. doi: 10.1101/gad.1432206.

Kondratova, Anna A., and Roman V. Kondratov. 2012. The circadian clock and pathology of the ageing brain. *Nature Reviews Neuroscience* 13 (5):325-335. doi: 10.1038/nrn 3208.

Kress, Geraldine J., Fan Liao, Julie Dimitry, Michelle R. Cedeno, Garret A. FitzGerald, David M. Holtzman, and Erik S. Musiek. 2018. Regulation of amyloid-β dynamics and pathology by the circadian clock. *Journal of Experimental Medicine, 215* (4):1059-1068. doi: 10.1084/jem.20172347.

Li, L., J. Xu, M. Wu, and J. M Hu. 2018. Protective role of microRNA-221 in Parkinson's disease. *Bratislava Medical Journal, 119* (01):22-27. doi: 10.4149/ bll_2018_005.

Liu, Elaine Y., Christopher P. Cali, and Edward B. Lee. 2017. RNA metabolism in neurodegenerative disease. *Disease Models & Mechanisms, 10* (5):509-518. doi: 10.1242/dmm.028613.

Lowrey, P. L., and J. S. Takahashi. 2004. Mammalian circadian biology: elucidating genome-wide levels of temporal organization. *Annual Review of Genomics and Human Genetics, 5*:407-41.doi:10.1146/annurev.genom.5.061903.175925.

Ma, Guoda, Yajun Wang, You Li, Lili Cui, Yujuan Zhao, Bin Zhao, and Keshen Li. 2015. MiR-206, a key modulator of skeletal muscle development and disease. *International Journal of Biological Sciences, 11* (3):345-352. doi: 10.7150/ijbs. 10921.

Matamala, José Manuel, Raul Arias-Carrasco, Carolina Sanchez, Markus Uhrig, Leslie Bargsted, Soledad Matus, Vinicius Maracaja-Coutinho, Sebastian Abarzua, Brigitte van Zundert, Renato Verdugo, Patricio Manque, and Claudio Hetz. 2018. Genome-wide circulating microRNA expression profiling reveals potential biomarkers for amyotrophic lateral sclerosis. *Neurobiology of Aging, 64*:123-138. doi:10.1016/j.neurobiolaging.2017.12.020.

Mendoza, J., and E. Challet. 2014. Circadian insights into dopamine mechanisms. *Neuroscience, 282*:230-242. doi: 10.1016/j.neuroscience.2014.07.081.

Nagaraj, Siranjeevi, Katarzyna Marta Zoltowska, Katarzyna Laskowska-Kaszub, and Urszula Wojda. 2019. microRNA diagnostic panel for Alzheimer's disease and epigenetic trade-off between neurodegeneration and cancer. *Ageing Research Reviews, 49*:125-143. doi: 10.1016/j.arr.2018.10.008.

Nguyen, Truyen, Paul Nioi, and Cecil B. Pickett. 2009. The Nrf2-antioxidant response element signaling pathway and its activation by oxidative stress. *Journal of Biological Chemistry, 284* (20):13291-13295. doi:10.1074/jbc.r900010200.

Niedzielska, Ewa, Irena Smaga, Maciej Gawlik, Andrzej Moniczewski, Piotr Stankowicz, Joanna Pera, and Małgorzata Filip. 2015. Oxidative Stress in neurodegenerative diseases. *Molecular Neurobiology, 53* (6):4094-4125. doi: 10.1007/s12035-015-93 37-5.

Patacchioli, F. R., P. Monnazzi, A. Scontrini, E. Tremante, I. Caridi, E. Brunetti, F. R. Buttarelli, and F. E. Pontieri. 2003. Adrenal dysregulation in amyotrophic lateral sclerosis. *Journal of Endocrinological Investigation, 26* (12):RC23-RC25. doi: 10.1007/bf03349149.

Piletič, Klara, and Tanja Kunej. 2016. MicroRNA epigenetic signatures in human disease. *Archives of Toxicology, 90* (10):2405-2419. doi: 10.1007/s00204016-1815-7.

Pivovarova, O., O. Gogebakan, S. Sucher, J. Groth, V. Murahovschi, K. Kessler, M. Osterhoff, N. Rudovich, A. Kramer, and A. F. Pfeiffer. 2016. Regulation of the clock gene expression in human adipose tissue by weight loss. *International Journal of Obesity*, *40* (6):899-906. doi: 10.1038/ijo.2016.34.

Preussner, M., and F. Heyd. 2016. Post-transcriptional control of the mammalian circadian clock: implications for health and disease. *Pflügers Archiv : European Journal of Physiology, 468* (6):983-91. doi: 10.1007/s00424-016-1820-y.

Raheja, Radhika, Keren Regev, Brian C. Healy, Maria Antonietta Mazzola, Vanessa Beynon, Felipe Von Glehn, Anu Paul, Camilo Diaz-Cruz, Taha Gholipour, Bonnie I. Glanz, Pia Kivisakk, Tanuja Chitnis, Howard L. Weiner, James D. Berry, and Roopali Gandhi. 2018. Correlating serum micrornas and clinical parameters in amyotrophic lateral sclerosis. *Muscle & Nerve*, *58* (2):261-269. doi: 10.1002/mus. 26106.

Renoux, Abigail J., and Peter K. Todd. 2012. Neurodegeneration the RNA way. *Progress in Neurobiology, 97* (2):173-189. doi:10.1016/j.pneurobio.2011.10.006.

Ricci, Claudia, Carlotta Marzocchi, and Stefania Battistini. 2018. MicroRNAs as biomarkers in amyotrophic lateral sclerosis. *Cells, 7* (11):219. doi:10.3390/ cells711 0219.

Roser, Anna Elisa, Lucas Caldi Gomes, Jonas Schünemann, Fabian Maass, and Paul Lingor. 2018. Circulating miRNAs as diagnostic biomarkers for Parkinson's disease. *Frontiers in Neuroscience, 12*. doi:10.3389/fnins.2018.00625.

Sarkar, S., E. B. Engler-Chiurazzi, J. Z. Cavendish, J. M. Povroznik, A. E. Russell, D. D. Quintana, P. H. Mathers, and J. W. Simpkins. 2019. Over-expression of miR-34a induces rapid cognitive impairment and Alzheimer's disease-like pathology. *Brain Research, 1721*:146327. doi:10.1016/j.brainres.2019.146327.

Sarkar, S., S. Jun, S. Rellick, D. D. Quintana, J. Z. Cavendish, and J. W. Simpkins. 2016. Expression of microRNA-34a in Alzheimer's disease brain targets genes linked to synaptic plasticity, energy metabolism, and resting state network activity. *Brain Research, 1646*:139-151. doi:10.1016/j.brainres.2016.05.026.

Saus, Ester, Virginia Soria, Geòrgia Escaramís, Francesca Vivarelli, José M. Crespo, Birgit Kagerbauer, José Manuel Menchón, Mikel Urretavizcaya, Mònica Gratacòs, and Xavier Estivill. 2010. Genetic variants and abnormal processing of pre-miR-182, a circadian clock modulator, in major depression patients with late insomnia. *Human Molecular Genetics, 19* (20):4017-4025. doi: 10.1093/hmg/ddq316.

Serafin, A., L. Foco, S. Zanigni, H. Blankenburg, A. Picard, A. Zanon, G. Giannini, I. Pichler, M. F. Facheris, P. Cortelli, P. P. Pramstaller, A. A. Hicks, F. S. Domingues, and C. Schwienbacher. 2015. Overexpression of blood microRNAs 103a, 30b, and 29a in L-dopa-treated patients with PD. *Neurology, 84* (7):645-653. doi: 10.1212/wnl.0000000000001258.

Sleipness, Evan P., Barbara A. Sorg, and Heiko T. Jansen. 2007. Diurnal differences in dopamine transporter and tyrosine hydroxylase levels in rat brain: dependence on the suprachiasmatic nucleus. *Brain Research, 1129*:34-42. doi: 10.1016/j.brainres.2006.10.063.

Smith, Pascal Y., Julia Hernandez-Rapp, Francis Jolivette, Cynthia Lecours, Kanchan Bisht, Claudia Goupil, Veronique Dorval, Sepideh Parsi, Françoise Morin, Emmanuel Planel, David A. Bennett, Francisco-Jose Fernandez-Gomez, Nicolas Sergeant, Luc Buée, Marie-Ève Tremblay, Frédéric Calon, and Sébastien S. Hébert. 2015. miR-132/212 deficiency impairs tau metabolism and promotes pathological aggregation in vivo. *Human Molecular Genetics, 24* (23):6721-6735. doi: 10.1093/ hmg/ddv377.

Stakos, Dimitrios A., Kimon Stamatelopoulos, Dimitrios Bampatsias, Marco Sachse, Eleftherios Zormpas, Nikolaos I. Vlachogiannis, Simon Tual-Chalot, and Konstantinos Stellos. 2020. The Alzheimer's disease amyloid-beta hypothesis in cardiovascular aging and disease. *Journal of the American College of Cardiology, 75* (8):952-967. doi: 10.1016/j.jacc.2019.12.033.

Swarbrick, S., N. Wragg, S. Ghosh, and Alexandra Stolzing. 2019. Systematic review of miRNA as biomarkers in Alzheimer's disease. *Molecular Neurobiology, 56* (9):6156-6167. doi: 10.1007/s12035-019-1500-y.

Tasca, Elisabetta, Valentina Pegoraro, Antonio Merico, and Corrado Angelini. 2016. Circulating microRNAs as biomarkers of muscle differentiation and atrophy in ALS. *Clinical Neuropathology, 35* (01):22-30. doi:10.5414/np300889.

Taylor, J. Paul, Robert H. Brown, and Don W. Cleveland. 2016. Decoding ALS: from genes to mechanism. *Nature, 539* (7628):197-206. doi:10.1038/nature20413.

Terrinoni, Alessandro, Cosimo Calabrese, Daniela Basso, Ada Aita, Sabrina Caporali, Mario Plebani, and Sergio Bernardini. 2018. The circulating miRNAs as diagnostic and prognostic markers. *Clinical Chemistry and Laboratory Medicine*, *57* (7):932-953. doi: 10.1515/cclm-2018-0838.

Tosches, M. A., D. Bucher, P. Vopalensky, and D. Arendt. 2014. Melatonin signaling controls circadian swimming behavior in marine zooplankton.*Cell, 159* (1):46-57. doi: 10.1016/j.cell.2014.07.042.

Tsang, Anthony H., Mariana Astiz, Brinja Leinweber, and Henrik Oster. 2017. Rodent models for the analysis of tissue clock function in metabolic rhythms research. *Frontiers in Endocrinology, 8*. doi: 10.3389/fendo.2017.00027.

Vallelunga, Annamaria, Tommaso Iannitti, Giovanna Dati, Sabrina Capece, Marco Maugeri, Ersilia Tocci, Marina Picillo, Giampiero Volpe, Autilia Cozzolino, Massimo

Squillante, Giulio Cicarelli, Paolo Barone, and Maria Teresa Pellecchia. 2019. Serum miR-30c-5p is a potential biomarker for multiple system atrophy. *Molecular Biology Reports, 46* (2):1661-1666. doi: 10.1007/s11033-019-04614-z.

Videnovic, Aleksandar, and Phyllis C. Zee. 2015. Consequences of circadian disruption on neurologic health. *Sleep Medicine Clinics, 10* (4):469-480.doi: 10.1016/j.jsmc.2015.08.004.

Wang, Qi, Svetlana N. Bozack, Yuanqing Yan, Michael E. Boulton, Maria B. Grant, and Julia V. Busik. 2014. Regulation of retinal inflammation by rhythmic expression of miR-146a in diabetic retina. *Investigative Opthalmology & Visual Science, 55* (6):3986. doi: 10.1167/iovs.13-13076.

Wang, Ruili, Ying Yang, Hui Wang, Ya He, and Chen Li. 2019. MiR-29c protects against inflammation and apoptosis in Parkinson's disease model in vivo and in vitro by targeting SP1. *Clinical and Experimental Pharmacology and Physiology, 47* (3):372-382. doi: 10.1111/1440-1681.13212.

Weigend, Susanne, Sebastian Holst, Josefine Meier, Matthias Brock, Malcolm Kohler, and Hans-Peter Landolt. 2018. Prolonged waking and recovery sleep affect the serum microRNA expression profile in humans. *Clocks & Sleep, 1* (1):75-87. doi: 10.3390/clockssleep1010008.

Wennstrom, M., and H. M. Nielsen. 2012. Cell adhesion molecules in Alzheimer's disease. *Degenerative Neurological and Neuromuscular Disease, 2*:65-77. doi: 10.2147/DNND.S19829.

West, A. C., and D. A. Bechtold. 2015. The cost of circadian desynchrony: evidence, insights and open questions. *Bioessays, 37* (7):777-88. doi:10.1002/bies.201400173.

Witkovsky, Paul. 2004. Dopamine and retinal function. *Documenta Ophthalmologica, 108* (1):17-39. doi: 10.1023/b:doop.0000019487.88486.0a.

Xia, Xiju, Xiaonan Fu, Binbin Wu, Jinsong Zhu, and Zhangwu Zhao. 2019. Circadian regulation of microRNA-target chimeras in Drosophila. *Cold Spring Harbor Laboratory.*

Zhou, Wei, Yan Li, Xia Wang, Lianqi Wu, and Yonghua Wang. 2011. MiR-206-mediated dynamic mechanism of the mammalian circadian clock. *BMC Systems Biology, 5* (1):141. doi: 10.1186/1752-0509-5-141.

Chapter 6

Application of Epigenetics in Neurological Disorders

Suyash Agarwal[1,*], Munmun Banerjee[2], Anurag Singh[2] and Jitendra Narayan[3,†]

[1]Redcliffe Life Tech Private Limited, Noida, India
[2]Amity Institute of Biotechnology, Amity University Uttar Pradesh, India
[3]CSIR-Institute of Genomics and Integrative Biology, Delhi, India

Abstract

According to emerging findings, epigenetic mechanisms are essential for the creation and maintenance of neural networks in the brain, as well as higher-order brain processes such as cognitive functions and behaviour. Defects in epigenetic pathways are now known to alter illness susceptibility, the aetiology or pathophysiology of numerous conditions, and treatment response. According to a large body of research, epigenetic dysfunctions have been linked to neurodevelopmental disorders such as Rett syndrome (RS), Fragile X syndrome, and Rubinstein-Taybi syndrome, as well as neurodegenerative and psychiatric conditions such as Alzheimer's disease (AD), frontotemporal lobar degeneration (FTLD), depression, and schizophrenia. Epigenetic pathways are also involved in the transgenerational impacts of the environment on brain and body functions, as well as the subsequent inheritance of disorders across generations.

This chapter investigates the function of dysregulated epigenetic pathways in the aetiology and pathophysiology of neurodevelopmental and neurodegenerative disorders using RS and AD as examples. It also

* Corresponding Author's Email: suyash.agarwal@redcliffelabs.com.
† Corresponding Author's Email: jnarayan@igib.res.in.

In: New Perspectives in Neuroscience
Editors: Prachi Srivastava, Neha Srivastava and Prekshi Garg
ISBN: 978-1-68507-754-9

explores the function of epigenetic mechanisms in the development of depression and their involvement in mediating antidepressant effects, highlighting the importance of the epigenome in psychiatric illnesses. The chapter finishes with a brief discussion of how early life trauma-induced epigenetic changes may impair adult brain functioning and how these effects are thought to be handed down through generations via epigenetic pathways.

Introduction

Neurological disorders are disorders of the nerve system. The worldwide toll of these illnesses is increasing. According to the Global Burden Disease Study 2015, Alzheimer's disease is one of the most frequent neurological disorders, accounting for nearly 10 million DALYs (Disability Adjusted Life Years) [1]. In the United States, Alzheimer's disease has been listed as one of the most burdensome neurological diseases in the Global Burden of Disease study of 2017 [2]. Since the nervous system acts like a "relay system" of the body, its impairment leads to an increased susceptibility to develop other diseases like cardiovascular diseases, metabolism-related diseases etc. [3]. The development of neurological illnesses cannot be traced back to a single factor, such as the genome, but must be traced back to a complex interplay of multiple variables that influence the genome. The regulation of the functioning of unmutated but modified DNA sequences and histones is known as epigenetics [4] and the altered genome is termed as epigenome. Epigenetics plays a major role in determining interaction of a gene with other genes as well as the environment which in turn impacts its expression [5]. The epigenome being dynamic varies with age [6], internal factors [7] and external environment [6]. Epigenetic mechanisms such as abnormalities, and disordered chromatin play a role in the pathogenesis of various neurological illnesses [6-8].

There is plenty of evidence to support the existence of epigenetic modifications in neurological disorders. Few studies suggest that the APP gene is hypomethylated in Alzheimer's disease [9] However, according to Sanchez-Mut et al., genes such as TBXA2R, F2RL2, SORBS3, and SPTBN4 are hypermethylated [10]. Frontotemporal lobar degeneration (FTLD) patients suffer from hypermethylation of CpG units in GRN promoter which negatively affects the transcription and translation of GRN gene [11]. In depression, genes like BDNF, NR3C1, PPFIA4 etc. depict altered patterns of methylation whereas histones vary in acetylation patterns [12]. Expression of a glycoprotein Reelin and a transcription factor SOX10 is also affected by methylation in case of schizophrenic patients [13]. Rett syndrome, which mostly affects females [14], is associated with defects in MECP2 (methyl-CpG binding protein 2) gene [15]. Another X-linked illness, fragile X syndrome, is connected with chromatin organisation flaws produced by FMRP depletion (fragile X syndrome retardation protein) [16]. Dysregulated lysine acetytransferase enzymes obstruct chromatin remodelling and can cause Rubinstein-Taybi syndrome [17].

Epigenetics when applied in the field of medicine has numerous applications. Epigenetic modifications in circulating nucleic acids [18] serve as efficient and stable biomarkers for diagnosing various neurological disorders [19]. Epigenomes can be inherited (transgenerational epigenetics) [20] like the genome which aids in forecasting the susceptibility of offspring to develop a particular medical condition. Detection of epigenetic modifications also leads to identification of pathways and parts of the nervous system involved in neurological disorders. Techniques for detection include methylation-sensitive digestion [21], whole genome bisulfite sequencing (WGBS), reduced representation bisulfite sequencing (RRBS) [22], methylated DNA immunoprecipitation (MeDIP), MNase (Micrococcal Nuclease) digestion followed by high-throughput sequencing, microarrays, chromatin immunoprecipitation (ChIP) assays etc. [23]. Epigenetic drift happens as we age, and epigenetic therapy could be a viable option for treating disease-causing changes caused by epigenetic drift [24]. This book chapter deals with various aspects of epigenetics that not only contribute to seven neurological disorders (Alzheimer's disease, FTLD, depression, schizophrenia, Rett syndrome, fragile X syndrome and Rubinstein-Taybi syndrome) but can also be applied for their therapy.

Neurological Disorders

Some epigenetic changes may differ amongst neurological illnesses, while others are ubiquitous. Several techniques are used for detection of epigenetic modifications. The most common techniques are the ones used to determine methylation patterns. Methylation sensitive digestion is one such technique that is carried out using Methylation Sensitive Restriction Enzyme (MSRE). MSRE cleaves DNA with unmethylated CpGs but has no effect on DNA with methylated CpGs. In the former case, Polymerase Chain Reaction (PCR) is disrupted as the DNA is fragmented but in the latter case, PCR proceeds normally [25]. Bisulfite conversion method relies on the difference in the ability of cytosine and 5mC (5-methylcytosine) to undergo deamination reaction. The inability of 5mC to get deaminated rapidly ensures that they retain their identity and are detected as 5mC in PCR. But cytosine is deaminated rapidly and at the end of bisulfite conversion process, it gets converted to uracil. During PCR, uracil is amplified as thymine. Here, PCR is performed as a part of sequencing [26]. In RRBS method, restriction fragments of DNA are subjected to bisulfite conversion process. These fragments are then amplified using PCR, cloned and finally sequenced to determine methylation status of DNA [27]. ChIP assays are based on immunoprecipitation. Treatment of a biological sample such as cells with formaldehyde causes fixation of cells by cross-linking protein and DNA. Cells are lysed to liberate the chromatin which is then fragmented. Exposure of these fragments to an antibody specific to a protein cross-linked to DNA causes immunoprecipitation of the protein-DNA complex. This is followed by de-cross-linking of DNA from the complex and its amplification through PCR for analysis of histone modifications [28]. MeDIP is another technique based on immunoprecipitation but it is only applicable for the detection of methylated DNA, particularly, 5mC. In MeDIP, genomic DNA is extracted from a biological sample, purified, fragmented and denatured. Anti-5-methylcytidine antibody is used for immunoprecipitation of methylated DNA [29, 30]. This can be further subjected to microarray analysis [29]. The property of MNase (in the presence of calcium ions) [31] to cleave 3'-5' phosphodiester bonds linking adjacent nucleotides in A-T rich regions [32] of DNA is exploited in MNase digestion method [31]. This approach is used to analyse chromatin abnormalities since MNase cleaves the linker DNA that connects adjacent nucleosomes, leaving the nucleosome core particle and the DNA wrapped around it intact. This DNA can be sequenced after it has been purified [33].

Neurodegenerative and Psychiatric Conditions

Alzheimer's Disease (AD)

AD is a neurodegenerative disorder characterized by amyloid plaque and neurofibrillary tangles (NFTs). Early Onset AD (EOAD) comprises cases of AD patients less than 61 years of age whereas Late Onset AD (LOAD) deals with the rest. The onset of pathogenesis is usually marked by brain damage produced by oxidative stress [34]. Amyloid plaques are particularly composed of (Aβ)42 isoform of amyloid-β (Aβ) peptide which is mainly formed through the amyloidogenic mechanism of APP processing. The presence of excess Aβ leads to neuronal deaths by activating apoptotic pathways [35, 36]. NFTs are composed of protein tau (hyperphosphorylated state) and formed in the cytoplasm of neurons in hippocampus and cortex regions [37]. Hindered transmission of nerve impulse leads to cognitive disablement [36]. Decreased cerebral blood flow is observed in AD patients [37]. APOE4 (ε4 allele of apolipoprotein E) is less efficient in Aβ clearance from the brain [38]. Along with aging and trisomy of chromosome 21 [37], it also serves as a risk factor for AD. Certain environmental factors may promote initiation and/or progression of AD by triggering epigenetic processes. Formaldehyde, in elevated levels, can lead to hyperphosphorylation of tau protein and may even promote cross-linking of Aβ molecules [39]. Few studies have stated about the existence of altered methylation patterns in genes ANK1, NEP, RPL13, CDH23, HOXA3 and BIN1 [40, 41]. CpG sites' methylation upstream of the promoter of NR3C1 in children has been associated with LOAD dementia [42]. Non-CpG methylation or hypomethylation of genes like PSEN1, APP, PP2A, S100A2 and CREB5 is linked to their overexpression while hyperphosphorylation of MTHER, APOE, SORB3, MAPT and Neprilysin switches off their expression. Demethylation of 5-methylcytosine is another factor in which decreased levels in various parts of the brain have been associated with late stage AD [41]. Acetylation events impacted during AD elicit in the form of low levels of H4K16Ac in brains of AD patients [43]. An increase in the levels of hippocampal HDAC2 and class II HDAC6 in the cortex and hippocampus, but a decrease in the levels of cortical SIRT1 (sirturin1) have been recorded [44]. The upregulation of HDAC6 and excess methylation of DDR1 (Discoidin Domain Receptor 1) have been associated with tau hyperphosphorylation and Aβ accumulation respectively [45]. In layer II of the entorhinal cortex, NFTs are attributed to neurons with low levels of DNMT1 (DNA methyltransferase 1). Amongst the microRNAs that are involved in the pathophysiology, miRNA-101 and miRNA-107 have attracted attention of researchers because their decreased levels lead to loss of regulated expression of APP and BACE-1 respectively, which contributes to their overexpression [44]. Promoters having high levels of H3 acetylation [45] and enhancer elements of Down syndrome cell adhesion molecule like 1 (DSCAML1) with low methylation are other factors for BACE1 overexpression [46].

Frontotemporal Lobar Degeneration (FTLD)

With heterogeneity in disease courses, FTLD is characterised by neurodegeneration of frontal and temporal lobes of the brain [47]. This incurable disorder arises because of deposition of either tau protein or transactive response DNA-binding protein 43. If tau inclusions are present, FTLD is identified as tauopathy. Else, it is identified as non-tauopathy [48]. Genetics accounts for the heritable nature of familial FTLD which is linked with mutations in genes like microtubule-associated tau (MAPT), progranulin (GRN), and chromosome 9 open reading frame 72 (C9orf72) [49]. Ventromedial prefrontal cortex (vmPFC) is more prone to FTLD [50]. In one of the studies conducted in 2018, it was observed that FTLD symptoms usually begin to appear at an age over 50 years [51]. Dysfunction of social cognition is one of the disabilities faced by patients. Personality changes are also common. Some also experience atrophy of cortex [50]. Patients usually speak less than normal. Gray matter density is decreased in the frontal region. Hypermethylation of GRN promoter is associated with FTLD. The presence of a promoter of C9orf72 gene in hypermethylated condition alleviates damage to neurons as well as degeneration of gray matter in frontal cortex [47] but marks a more aggressive disease course [52]. C9orf72 suffers a loss of function when there is low expression of C9orf72 mRNA due to erroneous transcripts produced by repeat-containing RNAs [53].

Depression

Depression develops as a result of chronic stress, sleeplessness, and a variety of other conditions. Recurrent stress leads to degeneration of hippocampal CA3 pyramidal neurons [54]. High levels of corticosteroids, low levels of BDNF (Brain-Derived Neurotrophic Factor) [55] and GABA (gamma-Aminobutyric acid) [56], glutamate toxicity [54], excess production of ROS and RNS [57], impaired synaptic transmission, lack of functional monoaminergic transmitters, altered receptors' sensitivity[58], low grade inflammatory state maintained for prolonged time with activated immune system etc. are some features associated with depression [57]. It has been observed in experiments that when cytokines like IL-1, IL-2 and IFN-α are administered, humans develop behavioral changes and other symptoms of depression [58]. In various studies, elevated levels of IL-6, IL-10, CRP (C-Reactive Protein), TNF-α and complement protein C3 have been reported in individuals suffering from depression [59]. Sometimes, hormonal imbalance such as problems with secretions of cortisol, melatonin, growth hormone, TSH (thyroid stimulating hormone) and prolactin may also lead to depression [60]. The norepinephrine (NE) and serotonin (5HT) systems don't function properly [61]. Sleep disturbances [62] and abnormal subgenual anterior cingulate cortex are observed.[63] In general, depression is marked by a rise in expression DNMTs and reduction in expression of DNA demethylases. Either of the promoters I and VI of BDNF are hypermethylated [64] while promoter KLF11 (Krüppel-like factor 11) is hypomethylated [65] in patients. Nucleus accumbens (NAc) shows elevated levels of DNMT3a but reduced levels of acetylated H3K14 [64]. Some genes which exist in hypomethylated condition in MDD (Major Depressive Disorder) include CAPRIN1 (Cell Cycle Associated Protein 1), CITED2 (cAMP-response element binding protein/p300-interacting transactivator with Glu/Asp-rich carboxy-terminal domain-2), DGKH (DiacylGlycerol Kinase), GSK3B (Glycogen Synthase Kinase 3 Beta) and SGK1 (Serum/Glucocorticoid Regulated Kinase 1) [66]. The peculiar acetylation pattern of H3K14, a drop in levels of HDAC2 in the NAc region and hike in HDAC2 mRNA levels in WBCs has been reported in MDD patients [67]. Hypomethylation of MET and its overexpression in cortex, hippocampus brain and frontal cortex regions has also been observed together with overexpression of HGF gene in cortex (BA24 region), frontal cortex as well as in whole blood. In people suffering from depression, mRNA levels of MET and HGF in the hippocampus deviate from normal levels and GABRA1 levels are low in the anterior prefrontal brain region. PSORS1C3 suffers from methylation problems in BA11 and BA25 regions of the brain. Altered DNA methylation patterns have been reported in GRIK2, ELOVL5 and BEGAIN genes in depressed patients committing suicide [68]. Overexpression of the ZBTB20 gene has also been recorded [69]. Absence of phosphorylated S421 MeCP2, methylation of H3 [67], reduction in expression of NR3C1 in HPA center and FKBP5 demethylation [66] are other contributing factors to depression.

Schizophrenia

Schizophrenia arises out of impaired communication among neurons. Transcription process for Myelin-Associated Glycoprotein (MAG), transferrin, 2´,3´-cyclic nucleotide 3´-phosphodiesterase (CNP) and quaking 1 is negatively impacted. Besides this, ADAM12 is altered. Certain genes are overexpressed like myelin-associated oligodendrocyte basic protein (MOBP), prohibitin, syntaxin binding protein 1 (STXBP1) and DISC1 (Disrupted in Schizophrenia 1). Lowered oligodendrocytes' density but increased density of astrocytes may be observed in different brain regions. Level of Glial Fibrillary Acidic Protein (GFAP) protein, expression of glutamine synthetase [70] and flow of blood in the prefrontal cortex is affected [71]. The NR1 subunit of AT-methyl-D-aspartate (NMDA) receptor has altered glycine binding site and may be overexpressed. Deficit of functional NR1 subunit is linked with dopamine activity problems in schizophrenia [72]. Overexpression of the NR2D subunit has also been reported [71]. Abnormal membrane structure and its dysfunction, Essential Fatty Acids (EFA), a drop in Poly-Unsaturated Fatty Acids (PUFAs) levels and elevated concentrations of Superoxide Dismutase (SOD) in RBC, malondialdehyde and pentane in blood, lipofuscin-like material depositions in oligodendrocyte [73] and low hippocampal synaptophysin concentration have been observed [74]. Oxidative as well as reductive stress contribute to redox imbalance and the free radicals so produced are routed to interrupt various cell signalling pathways [75]. All these factors including genetics [76] are responsible for development of symptoms peculiar to schizophrenia.

Several epigenetic processes are involved in schizophrenia. Increase in enzymes called DNMT1 and TET1 (ten-eleven translocase methylcytosine dioxygenase1) but decrease in the number of mRNA variants of BDNF has been seen in mice expressing schizophrenic behaviour after prenatal stress exposure. In humans suffering from the disease, BDNF mRNA and protein levels are low in the prefrontal cortex of the brain. There exists hypermethylation of promoters for genes RELN and GAD1 (Glutamic acid decarboxylase 1) whereas MB-COMT gene exists in hypomethylated condition [77]. RELN and SOX10 are downregulated [78]. Polymorphic 5-HT2A receptor (5-HT2AR) gene with C allele, is frequently observed in schizophrenic patients. It possesses such CpG sites which are capable of getting hypermethylated in patients. Other genes which are hypermethylated include CERS3, DPPA5, REC8, PRDM9, LY6G5C and DDX43. Some histone modifications include hypermethylation of PRDM9, low levels of acetylation of H3K9K14, low levels of HDAC2 [79] and high levels of HDac1. In the dorsolateral prefrontal cortex, H3K27ac levels are elevated in fetuses and infants inheriting schizophrenia [80]. NR3B and GRIA2 have been found hypomethylated in the frontal cortex portion of the brain while FOX2 is hypermethylated in parahippocampal gyrus and superior temporal gyrus. Some genes show gender-specific altered methylation patterns such as hypermethylation of MARLIN-1 in females and KCNJ6 in males. Some miRNAs (miR-132, miR-132-3p, miR-212, miR-544, miR-1307, miR-7 and miR-154-3p) that are known to be underexpressed in schizophrenic patients while miR-17 is overexpressed [81].

Neurodevelopmental Disorders

Rett Syndrome (RS)

This neurodevelopmental disorder is predominant in females as compared to males. This is because the MeCP2 gene which in mutated form significantly contributes to the development of this syndrome, is located on X-chromosome. Over 500 mutations in MeCP2 gene have been reported [82]. In fact, persons with the same mutation may experience varying levels of disease severity because of the phenomena of X-inactivation which itself takes place to variable extent amongst individuals [83]. RTT can be inherited in an X-linked dominant pattern and this happens in only 0.5% of the total RTT cases as majority of the cases (99.5%) are sporadic in nature [84]. Besides MeCP2, other genes that are known to contribute to development of syndrome include CDKL5 (cyclin-dependent kinase-like 5) and FOXG1 (forkhead box G1). There are chiefly three stages of RTT- onset, regression and plateau. Sometimes, a fourth stage characterised by motor deterioration is also considered [85]. Problems with brain development begin 6-18 months after the birth of an individual. Rett syndrome (RTT) patients experience breathing difficulties, sleep disturbances, scoliosis, gastrointestinal tract diseases, osteopenia [82] and apraxia [85]. Breathing problems are primarily grouped into two categories, namely, hyperventilation and breath-holding. In a study conducted by Tarquinio et al. in 2018, some patients also reported air-swallowing. In the same study, it was observed that breathing difficulties surface during early childhood itself in patients [86]. Gastrointestinal tract abnormalities include gastroesophageal reflux, bloating, gastroparesis, constipation. Though biliary tract disease is not common in RTT patients, it is lethal to those patients who develop this and currently, its incidence is rising. This disease has been usually identified in RTT females of older age and the ones with heredity of this disease [87]. Level of Cx3cr1 mRNA can get lowered in many parts of the brain as a consequence of RTT. Microglial cells may reduce in number [88]. Emotional, behavioural and autonomic dysregulation (EBAD) is observed in patients [89].

Fragile X Syndrome

Also known as Nonsyndromic Autism Spectrum Disorder, [90] this monogenic disorder caused by mutated Fragile X Mental Retardation-1 gene (FMR1) [91]. FMR1 gene suffers trinucleotide (CGG) repeat expansion and methylation at CpG dinucleotides, which is an epigenetic modification. When the number of this repeat in FMR1 allele ranges from 55 to 199, the allele is termed as premutation (PM) allele [92]. PM allele can convert into a fully mutated form in an individual only when the individual receives that allele from his mother [93]. FMR1 transcriptional start site is surrounded by a 3.8 kb long region which is hypermethylated [94]. Hypermethylation of the promoter [94] and H3 dimethylation [95] have been associated with silencing of genes. As a result of these biological events, the RNA-binding protein called Fragile X Mental Retardation Protein (FMRP) is either produced in low quantities or completely lacking which leads to fragile X syndrome [96]. Incidence of FXS in males and females is 1 in 5000 and 1 in 4000 to 8000 respectively [95]. FMRP is crucial for RNA biology, development of dendrites [97], regulating MBP and translation [98], potassium channels' activation, responding to DNA damage [95] and synaptic plasticity [99]. Dendritic development is affected in FXS because of lack of suppression of FMPR2-Cofilin pathway by FMRP which is deficient. Hikes in dendritic spine density with less spine maturity have been reported in cortex and hippocampus [100]. Proper cortical connectivity is absent [99] and size of caudate nucleus as well as lateral ventricles increases. Volume of frontal, temporal, parietal and occipital lobes is also impacted [100, 101]. Negative impact on GABA [100] and glutamatergic signaling [95] has been noticed. In astroglial cells, FMRP loss leads to reduction in mGluR5 receptors [102]. Oxidative stress in mitochondria is high and the antioxidant system malfunctions. ROS contributed by it to the brain may be considered as another reason for intellectual disability of patients [103]. Auditory hypersensitivity due to insufficient FMRP is observed in patients. Other symptoms include anxiety, language disorder, seizures, learning [97] and social deficits, mental retardation [104], distractibility [105], restricted [90] and reiterative behavior [106] and mitral valve prolapse [104]. The extent of mental retardation is usually greater in males as compared to females [107]. Sometimes, patients even suffer from autism simultaneously [106] because of the same mutated gene [105]. The physical appearance of patients is different from normal individuals and includes elongated face, wide forehead, large ears, extremely stretchable finger joints [100], abnormally high and narrow palate, pes planus, macroorchidism [104], dislocated joints. However, such characteristics are present in only patients with changes in connective tissue [95].

Rubinstein-Taybi Syndrome

Also known as broad thumb-hallux syndrome [108], this rare autosomal dominant disorder is mainly caused by abnormal CREBBP and EP300 genes. In the former case, it is categorised as RS type 1 while in the latter case, it is categorised as RS type 2 [109]. Incidence of this syndrome varies from 1 in 100,00 to 1 in 125,000 [110]. Development of cardiac complications in RS has been associated with loss of function mutation and polymorphism in ADCY9 (Adenylate cyclase type 9) gene [111]. Mental deficiency, speech impediments, visual impairment, seizures etc. are caused by failure of corpus callosum development [108]. Another set of complications experienced by RS patients are gastrointestinal disorders which include dysphagia, gastro-esophageal reflux, Hirschsprung disease and constipation [109]. Congenital malformations (cardiac, renal, spinal, ophthalmic) [112], facial deformities (eyebrows and palate arched greater than usual, long eyelashes, sloping palpebral fissures, crooked nose, wide nasal bridge, mandibular hypoplasia) [113] and respiratory infections are common to patients [114]. Behavioural disorders such as mood swings, inattentiveness, impulsivity, mental handicap etc. have also been observed. Abnormalities in hand and feet can be identified in patients and these encompass radial deviations of thumbs and halluces, widened fingers' phalanges, fetal finger pads tenacious even after birth and curved fifth finger [113]. Cardiac problems include septal defects, patent ductus arteriosus, stenosis, aortic coarctation, abnormalities in conduction, vascular rings etc. Ophthalmic complications include RT-associated infantile glaucoma, enophthalmos, degeneration of iris and optic nerve, nystagmus, crossed-eyes and high myopia [115]. Although many studies state that prenatal development of children with RT is normal, in a recent report, it has been stated that even prenatal growth may be hampered in some cases [116]. Slow growth leads to improper height and weight. At puberty, males are more likely to develop obesity earlier than females [117]. Patients are also susceptible to formation of various tumours [114].

Epigenetic Mechanism

The process of attaching a methyl group to the 5-position of a cytosine nucleotide, resulting in 5 methylcytosine (5-mC), is known as DNA methylation. For decades, scientists have known that there are considerable quantities of 5-mC in the genome, and research into 5-mC metabolism and control, DNA methylation-mediated gene-regulatory effects, and associated physiological activities has been continuing. As a result, these types of "methylomic" techniques are currently being used to investigate how genes are regulated in the nervous system, providing new insights into important neurobiologic processes like brain evolution, neural stem cell maintenance and differentiation, neurogenes etc.

The production of 5-mC is catalyse by members of the DNA methyltransferase (DNMT) family of enzymes, which use S-adenosyl-L-methionine as the methyl group donor for this biochemical reaction. DNMT3A and DNMT3B are principally engaged in de novo methylation, whereas DNMT1 is important in methylation maintenance by acting on hemimethylated DNA generated during DNA replication (i.e., a methylated parent strand with an unmethylated daughter strand). In the past, DNA methylation was assumed to be irreversible. However, it is now known that DNA methylation profiles are dynamic and vulnerable to demethylation, particularly in the brain [118].

NGS Based Applications in Epigenetics

Whole Genome Bisulfite Sequencing (WGBS)

Whole genome bisulfite sequencing (WGBS) is a next-generation sequencing technique that uses sodium bisulfite to detect the methylation status of single cytosines before sequencing. Unmethylated cytosines are converted to uracil by sodium bisulfite, a chemical molecule. Cytosines that do not convert to uracil are methylated. Unmethylated cytosines show as thymines after sequencing [119].

The widely used tool for methylation analysis is Bismark. Firstly, FASTQ files are quality-filtered and adapter contaminations trimmed using Trimmomatic. Secondly, a bisulfite-converted reference genome file is generated using Bowtie, and the epigenome sequence data is aligned on to the reference genome. Methylation information is mined from the *.sam file, and the output is utilized for visualization and reporting of downstream differential methylation calculations. There should be minimal bias as depicted in the M-bias plot in the methylation extraction report, which depicts the methylation percent across positions in the read. A perfectly horizontal line would represent an unbiased sequencing run. Integrative Genomics viewer (IGV) can be used for the visualization of methylated sites of the genome. The methylKit R package can be used for the calculation of differential methylation and homer can be used to annotate differentially methylated sites.

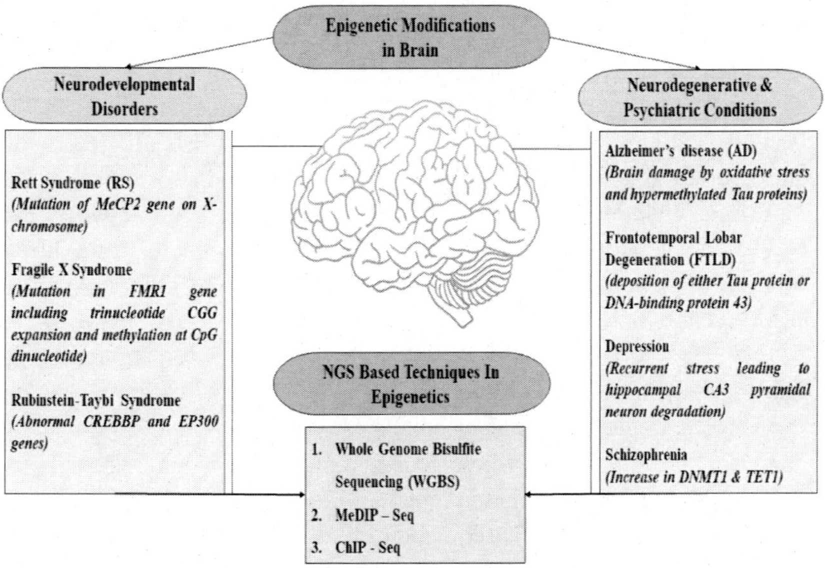

Figure 1. Diagrammatic representation of various neurodevelopmental and neurodegenerative disorders associated with epigenetic changes in the brain.

Advantages of Whole Genome Bisulfite Sequencing

- This technique is highly integrated single-base resolution DNA methylation patterning.
- It provides insights into reprogramming and gene cell-fate commitment, as well as gene regulation.
- It helps in the identification of novel epigenetic markers and targets for the disease.

MeDIP Sequencing (MeDIP-Seq)

MeDIP-seq is a NGS application which combines methylated DNA immunoprecipitation with the next-generation sequencing to carry out epigenetic studies at the genome-wide levels or at any specific regions of interest. MeDIP can detect methylated cytosines in mC and mCG contexts, and possibly hmC, 5-formylcytosine, and 5-carboxylcytosine as well. MeDIP-seq makes use of anti-5-methylcytosine antibodies coupled to magnetic beads to select for genomic fragments that are methylated. The fragments obtained are sequenced using Illumina and the read coverage can be a parameter, which could be used to estimate the methylation level of the region that they map to. The genome-wide 5-hydroxymethylcytosine (hmC) can also be detected by making use of a hydroxymethylated DNA immunoprecipitation (hMeDIP) procedure coupled with a 5hmC-specific antibody. MeDIP-seq neither requires uracil-tolerant DNA polymerase nor it introduces any mutations. MeDIP-seq technology is widely used to profile genome-wide DNA methylation when low amounts of DNA samples are available. It provides the resolution of several hundred base pairs in minimal selection bias and at a competitive cost.

Advantages of MeDIP Sequencing

- It can target mCG, mC or hmC
- It can be applied to whole genome or any regions of interest
- It is near-unbiased and hypothesis
- It helps in Epigenetic biomarker discovery
- It provides single-nucleotide resolution and is cost-effective
- Low input DNA requirement

ChIP-Seq

ChIP-Seq (chromatin immunoprecipitation sequencing), refers to the binding site analysis, is a way to analyze DNA-protein interactions. The technique combines NGS with chromatin immunoprecipitation (ChIP) to decipher where the DNA binds to the associated proteins. It can be used to reveal the binding sites of any protein of interest throughout the genome. ChIP-seq is often used to figure out how chromatin-related proteins and other transcription factors affect phenotypic mechanisms. Determining how proteins interact with DNA to regulate gene expression is essential to fully understand many biological processes and disease states. ChIP-Seq is a widely used tool to discern and quantify the specific DNA sequences where proteins bind or epigenetic modifications exist. This technology has played valuable roles in applications including studies on gene regulation, transcription complex assembly, DNA repair, histone modification, developmental mechanisms, disease progression and modifications.

Advantages of ChIP-Seq

- Exceptionally high-resolution and high quality sequencing: Millions of sequence tags can be obtained along with rare protein binding sites in the genome; it has the ability to mine novel enrichment sites.
- Cost-effective technique: efficient and rapid genome-wide profiling using multiple samples in one run and only using 1/100 of the amount of DNA required for ChIP-chip.
- Comprehensive analysis: Utilizing widely accepted software and latest programs for peak annotation, motif prediction, data visualization and functional analysis of ChIP-Seq.

Conclusion

The epigenetic community is rapidly focusing on the combined NGS with established DNA methylation capture methods, which would enable the improvement of the methylome analysis in context to neurological disorders and various other sectors . Hence, in the last few years, NGS based techniques have seen a boom and became an effective tool for DNA methylation profiling at a single-base level and at relatively affordable price. Furthermore, the involvement of NGS has significantly contributed to the increased knowledge on deciphering the differentially methylated DNA regions and the discovery of novel gene regulatory elements associated with the epigenetic machinery. These massive-parallel technologies provide great strength to decode the patterns and nature of DNA modifications, as well as their implications in the various physiologic and pathologic processes.

References

[1] GBD 2016 Neurology Collaborators. Global, regional, and national burden of neurological disorders, 1990-2016: a systematic analysis for the global burden of

disease study 2016. *Lancet Neurology*. [internet]. 2019 May [cited 2021 Sept 9]; 18(5):459-480. Available from: https://www.ncbi.nl m.nih.gov/pmc/articles/PMC6 459001/.

[2] GBD 2017 US Neurological Disorders Collaborators, Feigin VL, Vos T, Alahdab F, Amit AML, Bärnighausen TW, Beghi E, Beheshti M, Chavan PP, Criqui MH, Desai R, Dhamminda Dharmaratne S, Dorsey ER, Wilder Eagan A, Elgendy IY, Filip I, Giampaoli S, Giussani G, Hafezi-Nejad N, Hole MK, Ikeda T, Owens Johnson C, Kalani R, Khatab K, Khubchandani J, Kim D, Koroshetz WJ, Krishnamoorthy V, Krishnamurthi RV, Liu X, Lo WD, Logroscino G, Mensah GA, Miller TR, Mohammed S, Mokdad AH, Moradi-Lakeh M, Morrison SD, Shivamurthy VKN, Naghavi M, Nichols E, Norrving B, Odell CM, Pupillo E, Radfar A, Roth GA, Shafieesabet A, Sheikh A, Sheikhbahaei S, Shin JI, Singh JA, Steiner TJ, Stovner LJ, Wallin MT, Weiss J, Wu C, Zunt JR, Adelson JD, Murray CJL. Burden of neurological disorders across the US from 1990-2017: a global burden of disease study. *JAMA Neurol*. [internet]. 2021 Feb 1 [cited 2021 Sept 9]; 78(2):165-176. Available from: https://www.ncbi.nlm.nih.gov/pmc/articles/PMC 7607495/.

[3] Hoffmann A, Sportelli V, Ziller M, Spengler D. Epigenomics of major depressive disorders and schizophrenia: early life decides. *International Journal of Molecular Sciences.* [internet]. 2017 Aug 4 [cited 2021 Sept 9];18(8):1711. Available from: https://www.ncbi.nlm.nih.gov/pmc/articles/PMC5578101/.

[4] Ptak C, Petronis A. Epigenetic approaches to psychiatric disorders. *Dialogues in Clinical Neuroscience* [internet]. 2010 [cited 2021 Sept 9];12(1):25-35. Available from: https://www.ncbi.nlm.nih.gov/pmc/articles/PMC3181944/.

[5] Qureshi IA, Mehler MF. Advances in epigenetics and epigenomics for neurodegenerative diseases. *Current Neurology and Neuroscience Reports* [internet]. 2011 Oct [cited 2021 Sept 9];11(5):464-73. Available from: https://www.ncbi.nlm.nih.gov/pmc/articles/PMC4461866/.

[6] Delgado-Morales R, Agís-Balboa R, Esteller M. et al. Epigenetic mechanisms during ageing and neurogenesis as novel therapeutic avenues in human brain disorders. *Clinical Epigenetics* [internet]. 2017 [cited 2021 Sept 9]; 9:67. Available from: https://link.springer.com/article/10.1186/s13148-017-0365-z#citeas/.

[7] Kanherkar RR, Bhatia-Dey N, Csoka AB. Epigenetics across the human lifespan. *Frontiers in Cell and Developmental Biology* [internet]. 2014 Sep 9 [cited 2021 Sept 9];2:49. Available from: https://www.ncbi.nlm.nih.gov/pmc/articles/PMC 4207041/.

[8] Jakovcevski M, Akbarian S. Epigenetic mechanisms in neurological disease. *Nature Medicine* [internet]. 2012 Aug [cited 2021 Sept 9];18(8):1194-204. Available from: https://www.ncbi.nlm.nih.gov/pmc/articles/PMC3596876/.

[9] Xiao X, Liu X, Jiao B. Epigenetics: recent advances and its role in the treatment of Alzheimer's disease. *Frontiers in Neurology* [internet]. 2020 Oct 15 [cited 2021 Sept 9];11:538301. Available from: https://www.ncbi.nlm.nih.gov/pmc/articles/P MC7594522/.

[10] Sanchez-Mut JV, Aso E, Panayotis N, Lott I, Dierssen M, Rabano A, Urdinguio RG, Fernandez AF, Astudillo A, Martin-Subero JI, Balint B, Fraga MF, Gomez A,

Gurnot C, Roux JC, Avila J, Hensch TK, Ferrer I, Esteller M. DNA methylation map of mouse and human brain identifies target genes in Alzheimer's disease. *Brain* [internet]. 2013 Oct [cited 2021 Sept 9];136(Pt 10):3018-27. Available from: https://www.ncbi.nlm.nih.gov/pmc/articles/PMC3784285/.

[11] Banzhaf-Strathmann J, Claus R, Mücke O, Rentzsch K, van der Zee J, Engelborghs S, De Deyn PP, Cruts M, van Broeckhoven C, Plass C, Edbauer D. Promoter DNA methylation regulates progranulin expression and is altered in FTLD. *Acta Neuropathologica Communications* [internet]. 2013 May 13 [cited 2021 Sept 9];1:16. Available from: https://www.ncbi.nlm.nih.gov/pmc/articles/PMC38935 57/.

[12] Czarny P, Białek K, Ziółkowska S, Strycharz J, Barszczewska G, Sliwinski T. The importance of epigenetics in diagnostics and treatment of major depressive disorder. *Journal of Personalized Medicine* [internet]. 2021 Mar 1 [cited 2021 Sept 9];11(3):167. Available from: https://www.ncbi.nlm.nih.gov/pmc/articles/PMC7 999864/.

[13] Rajarajan P, Jiang Y, Kassim BS, Akbarian S. Chromosomal conformations and epigenomic regulation in schizophrenia. *Progress in Molecular Biology and Translational Science*. [internet]. 2018 [cited 2021 Sept 9];157:21-40. Available from: https://www.ncbi.nlm.nih.gov/pmc/articles/PMC6318347/.

[14] Ehrhart F, Coort SL, Cirillo E, Smeets E, Evelo CT, Curfs LM. Rett syndrome - biological pathways leading from MECP2 to disorder phenotypes. *Orphanet Journal of Rare Diseases* [internet]. 2016 Nov 25 [cited 2021 Sept 9];11(1):158. Available from: https://www.ncbi.nlm.nih.gov/pmc/articles/PMC5123333/.

[15] Liyanage VR, Rastegar M. Rett syndrome and MeCP2. *NeuroMolecular Medicine* [internet]. 2014 Jun [cited 2021 Sept 9];16(2):231-64. Available from: https://www.ncbi.nlm.nih.gov/pmc/articles/PMC5798978/.

[16] Dionne O, Corbin F. An *omic* overview of fragile x syndrome. *Biology* (Basel) [internet]. 2021 May 13 [cited 2021 Sept 9];10(5):433. Available from: https://www.ncbi.nlm.nih.gov/pmc/articles/PMC8153138/.

[17] Gils J, Magdinier F, Fergelot P, Lacombe D. Rubinstein-Taybi syndrome: a model of epigenetic disorder. *Genes* (Basel) [internet]. 2021 Jun 24 [cited 2021 Sept 9];12(7):968. Available from: https://www.ncbi.nlm.nih.gov/pmc/articles/PMC8 30 3114/.

[18] Bruno DCF, Donatti A, Martin M, Almeida VS, Geraldis JC, Oliveira FS, Dogini DB, Lopes-Cendes I. Circulating nucleic acids in the plasma and serum as potential biomarkers in neurological disorders. *Brazilian Journal of Medical and Biological Research* [internet]. 2020 [cited 2021 Sept 9];53(10):e9881. Available from: https://www.ncbi.nlm.nih.gov/pmc/articles/PMC7446710/.

[19] Chung FF, Herceg Z. The promises and challenges of toxico-epigenomics: environmental chemicals and their impacts on the epigenome. *Environ Health Perspect* [internet]. 2020 Jan [cited 2021 Sept 9];128(1):15001. Available from: https://www.ncbi.nlm.nih.gov/pmc/articles/PMC7015548/.

[20] Burggren W. Epigenetic inheritance and its role in evolutionary biology: re-evaluation and new perspectives. *Biology* (Basel) [internet]. 2016 May 25 [cited

2021 Sept 9];5(2):24. Available from: https://www.ncbi.nlm.nih.gov/pmc/articles/PMC4929538/.

[21] Han Y, Garcia BA. Combining genomic and proteomic approaches for epigenetics research. *Epigenomics* [internet]. 2013 Aug [cited 2021 Sept 9];5(4):439-52. Available from: https://www.ncbi.nlm.nih.gov/pmc/articles/PMC4055025/.

[22] Angrish MM, Allard P, McCullough SD, Druwe IL, Helbling Chadwick L, Hines E, Chorley BN. Epigenetic Applications in adverse outcome pathways and environmental risk evaluation. *Environmental Health Perspectives*. [internet]. 2018 Apr 12 [cited 2021 Sept 9];126(4):045001. Available from: https://www.ncbi.nlm.nih.gov/pmc/articles/PMC6071815/.

[23] Xu Y, Doonan SR, Ordog T, Bailey RC. Translational opportunities for microfluidic technologies to enable precision epigenomics. *Analytical Chemistry* [internet]. 2020 Jun 16 [cited 2021 Sept 10];92(12):7989-7997. Available from: https://www.ncbi.nlm.nih.gov/pmc/articles/PMC8053002/.

[24] Li Y, Tollefsbol TO. Age-related epigenetic drift and phenotypic plasticity loss: implications in prevention of age-related human diseases. *Epigenomics* [internet]. 2016 Dec [cited 2021 Sept 10];8(12):1637-1651. Available from: https://www.ncbi.nlm.nih.gov/pmc/articles/PMC5618938/.

[25] Hashimoto K, Kokubun S, Itoi E, Roach HI. Improved quantification of DNA methylation using methylation-sensitive restriction enzymes and real-time PCR. *Epigenetics* [internet]. 2007 Apr-Jun [cited 2021 Sept 10];2(2):86-91. Available from: https://www.tandfonline.com/doi/abs/10.4161/epi.2.2.4203/.

[26] Martisova A, Holcakova J, Izadi N, Sebuyoya R, Hrstka R, Bartosik M. DNA methylation in Solid Tumors: Functions and Methods of Detection. *Int J Mol Sci*. [internet]. 2021 Apr 19 [cited 2021 Sept 10];22(8):4247. Available from: https://www.ncbi.nlm.nih.gov/pmc/articles/PMC8073724/.

[27] Meissner A, Gnirke A, Bell GW, Ramsahoye B, Lander ES, Jaenisch R. Reduced representation bisulfite sequencing for comparative high-resolution DNA methylation analysis. *Nucleic Acids Research*. [internet]. 2005 Oct 13 [cited 2021 Sept 10];33(18):5868-77. Available from: https://www.ncbi.nlm.nih.gov/pmc/articles/PMC1258174/.

[28] Pillai S, Chellappan SP. ChIP on chip assays: genome-wide analysis of transcription factor binding and histone modifications. *Methods in Molecular Biology* [internet]. 2009 [cited 2021 Sept 10];523:341-66. Available from: https://link.springer.com/protocol/10.1007%2F978-159745-190-1_23/.

[29] Weng YI, Huang TH, Yan PS. Methylated DNA immunoprecipitation and microarray-based analysis: detection of DNA methylation in breast cancer cell lines. *Methods in Molecular Biology* [internet]. 2009 [cited 2021 Sept 10];590:165-76. Available from: https://www.ncbi.nlm.nih.gov/pmc/articles/PMC2845920/.

[30] Weng YI, Huang TH, Yan PS. Methylated DNA immunoprecipitation and microarray-based analysis: detection of DNA methylation in breast cancer cell lines. *Methods in Molecular Biology*. [internet]. 2009 [cited 2021 Sept 10];590:165-76. Available from: https://www.ncbi.nlm.nih.gov/pmc/articles/PMC2845920/.

[31] Chereji RV, Bryson TD, Henikoff S. Quantitative MNase-seq accurately maps nucleosome occupancy levels. *Genome Biology*. [internet]. 2019 Sep 13 [cited 2021 Sept 10];20(1):198. Available from: https://www.ncbi.nlm.nih.gov/pmc/articles/PMC6743174/.

[32] Dingwall C, Lomonossoff GP, Laskey RA. High sequence specificity of micrococcal nuclease. *Nucleic Acids Research.* [internet]. 1981 Jun 25 [cited 2021 Sept 10];9(12):2659-73. Available from: https://www.ncbi.nlm.nih.gov/pmc/articles/PMC326883/.

[33] Voong LN, Xi L, Wang JP, Wang X. Genome-wide mapping of the nucleosome landscape by micrococcal nuclease and chemical mapping. *Trends in Genetics.* [internet]. 2017 Aug [cited 2021 Sept 10];33(8):495-507. Available from: https://www.ncbi.nlm.nih.gov/pmc/articles/PMC5536840/.

[34] Polis B, Samson AO. A new perspective on Alzheimer's disease as a brain expression of a complex metabolic disorder. in: Wisniewski T, editor. *Alzheimer's Disease* [ebook]. Brisbane: Codon Publications; 2019. p. 1-28. Available from: https://www.ncbi.nlm.nih.gov/books/NBK552149/ [cited 2021 Sept 10].

[35] Solis E Jr, Hascup KN, Hascup ER. Alzheimer's disease: the link between amyloid-β and neurovascular dysfunction. *Journal of Alzheimer's Disease*. [internet]. 2020 [cited 2021 Sept 10];76(4):1179-1198. Available from: https://www.ncbi.nlm.nih.gov/pmc/articles/PMC7483596/.

[36] Zuo L, Hemmelgarn BT, Chuang CC, Best TM. The role of oxidative stress-induced epigenetic alterations in amyloid-β production in Alzheimer's disease. *Oxidative Medicine and Cellular Longevity* [internet]. 2015 [cited 2021 Sept 10];2015:604658. Available from: https://www.ncbi.nlm.nih.gov/pmc/articles/PMC4620382/.

[37] Kumar A, Sidhu J, Goyal A, et al. Alzheimer disease. [Updated 2021 Aug 11]. In: *StatPearls* [ebook]. Treasure Island (FL): StatPearls Publishing. 2021 Jan. Available from: https://www.ncbi.nlm.nih.gov/books/NBK499922/ [cited 2021 Sept 10].

[38] Yamazaki Y, Zhao N, Caulfield TR, Liu CC, Bu G. Apolipoprotein E and Alzheimer disease: pathobiology and targeting strategies. *Nature Reviews Neurology*. [internet]. 2019 Sep [cited 2021 Sept 10];15(9):501-518. Available from: https://www.ncbi.nlm.nih.gov/pmc/articles/PMC7055192/.

[39] Wang F, Chen D, Wu P, Klein C, Jin C. Formaldehyde, Epigenetics, and Alzheimer's disease. *Chemical Research in Toxicology*. [internet]. 2019 May 20 [cited 2021 Sept 10];32(5):820-830. Available from: https://www.ncbi.nlm.nih.gov/pmc/articles/PMC6878761/.

[40] Gasparoni G, Bultmann S, Lutsik P, Kraus TFJ, Sordon S, Vlcek J, Dietinger V, Steinmaurer M, Haider M, Mulholland CB, Arzberger T, Roeber S, Riemenschneider M, Kretzschmar HA, Giese A, Leonhardt H, Walter J. DNA methylation analysis on purified neurons and glia dissects age and Alzheimer's disease-specific changes in the human cortex. *Epigenetics and Chromatin.* [internet]. 2018 Jul 25 [cited 2021 Sept 10];11(1):41. Available from: https://www.ncbi.nlm.nih.gov/pmc/articles/PMC6058387/.

[41] Atlante A, Amadoro G, Bobba A, Latina V. Functional foods: an approach to modulate molecular mechanisms of Alzheimer's disease. *Cells* [internet]. 2020 Oct 23 [cited 2021 Sept 11];9(11):2347. Available from: https://www.mdpi.com/2073-4409/9/11/2347/.

[42] Lemche E. Early Life Stress and Epigenetics in late-onset Alzheimer's dementia: a systematic review. *Current Genomics* [internet]. 2018 Nov [cited 2021 Sept 11];19(7):522-602. Available from: https://www.ncbi.nlm.nih.gov/pmc/articles/PMC6194433/.

[43] Tecalco-Cruz AC, Ramírez-Jarquín JO, Alvarez-Sánchez ME, Zepeda-Cervantes J. Epigenetic basis of Alzheimer disease. *World Journal of Biological Chemistry*. [internet]. 2020 Sep 27 [cited 2021 Sept 11];11(2):62-75. Available from: https://www.ncbi.nlm.nih.gov/pmc/articles/PMC7520642/.

[44] Adwan L, Zawia NH. Epigenetics: a novel therapeutic approach for the treatment of Alzheimer's disease. *Pharmacology and Therapeutics*. [internet]. 2013 Jul [cited 2021 Sept 11];139(1):41-50. Available from: https://www.ncbi.nlm.nih.gov/pmc/articles/PMC3693222/.

[45] Veerappan CS, Sleiman S, Coppola G. Epigenetics of Alzheimer's disease and frontotemporal dementia. *Neurotherapeutics* [internet]. 2013 Oct [cited 2021 Sept 11];10(4):709-21. Available from: https://www.ncbi.nlm.nih.gov/pmc/articles/PMC3805876/.

[46] Balmik AA, Chinnathambi S. Methylation as a key regulator of Tau aggregation and neuronal health in Alzheimer's disease. *Cell Commucation and Signaling*. [internet]. 2021 May 7 [cited 2021 Sept 11];19(1):51. Available from: https://www.ncbi.nlm.nih.gov/pmc/articles/PMC8103764/.

[47] Placek K, Massimo L, Olm C, Ternes K, Firn K, Van Deerlin V, Lee EB, Trojanowski JQ, Lee VM, Irwin D, Grossman M, McMillan CT. Cognitive reserve in frontotemporal degeneration: Neuroanatomic and neuropsychological evidence. *Neurology* [internet]. 2016 Oct 25 [cited 2021 Sept 11];87(17):1813-1819. Available from: https://www.ncbi.nlm.nih.gov/pmc/articles/PMC5089523/.

[48] Kumar-Singh S, Van Broeckhoven C. Frontotemporal lobar degeneration: current concepts in the light of recent advances. *Brain Patholo*gy [internet]. 2007 Jan [cited 2021 Sept 11];17(1):104-14. Available from: https://www.ncbi.nlm.nih.gov/pmc/articles/PMC8095552/.

[49] Olney NT, Ong E, Goh SM, Bajorek L, Dever R, Staffaroni AM, Cobigo Y, Bock M, Chiang K, Ljubenkov P, Kornak J, Heuer HW, Wang P, Rascovsky K, Wolf A, Appleby B, Bove J, Bordelon Y, Brannelly P, Brushaber D, Caso C, Coppola G, Dickerson BC, Dickinson S, Domoto-Reilly K, Faber K, Ferrall J, Fields J, Fishman A, Fong J, Foroud T, Forsberg LK, Gearhart DJ, Ghazanfari B, Ghoshal N, Goldman J, Graff-Radford J, Graff-Radford NR, Grant I, Grossman M, Haley D, Hsiung G, Huey ED, Irwin DJ, Jones DT, Kantarci K, Karydas AM, Kaufer D, Kerwin D, Knopman DS, Kramer JH, Kraft R, Kremers W, Kukull W, Lapid MI, Litvan I, Mackenzie IR, Maldonado M, Manoochehri M, McGinnis SM, McKinley EC, Mendez MF, Miller BL, Onyike C, Pantelyat A, Pearlman R, Petrucelli L, Potter M, Rademakers R, Ramos EM, Rankin KP, Roberson ED, Rogalski E, Sengdy P, Shaw LM, Syrjanen J, Tartaglia MC, Tatton N, Taylor J, Toga A,

Trojanowski JQ, Weintraub S, Wong B, Wszolek Z, Boxer AL, Boeve BF, Rosen HJ; Clinical and volumetric changes with increasing functional impairment in familial frontotemporal lobar degeneration. *Alzheimers & Dementia.* [internet]. 2020 Jan [cited 2021 Sept 11];16(1):49-59. Available from: https://www.ncbi.nlm.nih.gov/pmc/articles/PMC6988137/.

[50] Grossman M, Eslinger PJ, Troiani V, Anderson C, Avants B, Gee JC, McMillan C, Massimo L, Khan A, Antani S. The role of ventral medial prefrontal cortex in social decisions: converging evidence from fMRI and frontotemporal lobar degeneration. *Neuropsychologia* [internet].2010 Oct [cited 2021 Sept 11];48(12):3505-12. Available from: https://www.ncbi.nlm.nih.gov/pmc/articles/PMC2949451/.

[51] Forrest SL, Halliday GM, McCann H, McGeachie AB, McGinley CV, Hodges JR, Piguet O, Kwok JB, Spillantini MG, Kril JJ. Heritability in frontotemporal tauopathies. *Alzheimers & Dementia* [internet]. 2019 Jan 24 [cited 2021 Sept 15];11:115-124. Available from: https://www.ncbi.nlm.nih.gov/pmc/articles/PMC6351353/.

[52] Braems E, Swinnen B, Van Den Bosch L. C9orf72 loss-of-function: a trivial, stand-alone or additive mechanism in C9 ALS/FTD? *Acta Neuropathologica.* [internet]. 2020 Nov [cited 2021 Sept 15];140(5):625-643. Available from: https://www.ncbi.nlm.nih.gov/pmc/articles/PMC7547039/.

[53] Gendron TF, Belzil VV, Zhang YJ, Petrucelli L. Mechanisms of toxicity in C9FTLD/ALS. *Acta Neuropathologica.* [internet]. 2014 Mar [cited 2021 Sept 15];127(3):359-76. Available from: https://www.ncbi.nlm.nih.gov/pmc/articles/PMC4002260/.

[54] Duman RS. Pathophysiology of depression: the concept of synaptic plasticity. *European Psychiatry*. [internet] 2002 Jul [cited 2021 Sept 15];17 Suppl 3:306-10. Available from: http://citeseerx.ist.psu.edu/viewdoc/download?doi=10.1.1.1046.2494&rep=rep1&type=pdf/.

[55] Hacimusalar Y, Eşel E. Suggested Biomarkers for major depressive disorder. *Archives of Neuropsychiatry*. [internet]. 2018 May 28 [cited 2021 Sept 15];55(3):280-290. Available from: https://www.ncbi.nlm.nih.gov/pmc/articles/PMC6138223/.

[56] Bains N, Abdijadid S. Major depressive disorder. [updated 2021 Apr 20]. In: *StatPearls* [ebook]. Treasure Island (FL): StatPearls Publishing; 2021 Jan. Available from: https://www.ncbi.nlm.nih.gov/books/NBK559078/#_NBK559078_pubdet_/ [cited 2021 Sept 15].

[57] Carvalho AF, Miskowiak KK, Hyphantis TN, Kohler CA, Alves GS, Bortolato B, G Sales PM, Machado-Vieira R, Berk M, McIntyre RS. Cognitive dysfunction in depression - pathophysiology and novel targets. *CNS and Neurological Disorders - Drug Targets* [internet]. 2014 [cited 2021 Sept 15];13(10):1819-35. Available from: https://www.researchgate.net/publication/269189462_Cognitive_Dysfunction_in_Depression_-_Pathophysiology_and_Novel_Targets/.

[58] Brigitta B. Pathophysiology of depression and mechanisms of treatment. *Dialogues in Clinical Neuroscience.* [internet]. 2002 Mar [cited 2021 Sept 15];4(1):7-20. Available from: https://www.ncbi.nlm.nih.gov/pmc/articles/PMC3181668/.

[59] Nobis A, Zalewski D, Waszkiewicz N. Peripheral markers of depression. *Journal of Clincial Medicine* [internet]. 2020 Nov 24 [cited 2021 Sept 15];9(12):3793. Available from: https://www.ncbi.nlm.nih.gov/pmc/articles/PMC7760788/.

[60] Bernaras E, Jaureguizar J, Garaigordobil M. Child and adolescent depression: a review of theories, evaluation instruments, prevention programs, and treatments. *Frontiers in Psychology*. [internet]. 2019 Mar 20 [cited 2021 Sept 15];10:543. Available from: https://www.frontiersin.org/articles/10.3389/fpsyg.2019.00543/full/.

[61] Nemeroff CB. More than one-half of a decade of experience with venlafaxine dual serotonin-norepinephrine reuptake inhibitor. *Depression and Anxiety* [internet]; 2000 [cited 2021 Sept 15]; 12. Available from: https://policymed.typepad.com/files/depression-and-anexity-supplement---nemeroff-article-2000.pdf/.

[62] Srinivasan V, Pandi-Perumal SR, Trakht I, Spence DW, Hardeland R, Poeggeler B, Cardinali DP. Pathophysiology of depression: role of sleep and the melatonergic system. *Psychiatry Research*. [internet]. 2009 Feb 28 [cited 2021 Sept 15];165(3):201-14. Available from: https://d1wqtxts1xzle7.cloudfront.net/49514161/Role_of_melatonin_in_neurodegenerative_d20161010-8616-13z6gxc-with-cover-pagev2.pdf?Expires=1635883319&Signature=XpdOM3ManMQ68fUWXBsAv-3kSq54nKJdpO4EH3q0RGQRyNQskPMRhecHavuB-Cr2gIn3w~CG6Q1KljFWAY7KbXItMy-UagsXaABKg54yRHV-hvbfEN-OBCq2jDNLsT91HnBr~QJZLaY~ibfb1CmaOOb8VWxGp9zZ6IO~EWo~Mjsh2RqWIPjfa9PmNVBvldNdCxEDjr4fXXppk9mhQKV1JLQ2Qe1AMRG8EZWVg3F4UOiAXF8-iYboi1ukg4v5cwNqP9sA5CqwOh6PtIdHrRsIq2rUCsPR4ZiWzvH5tA~BhI7FYZ65BEnCPdBrBQwUUn2X~lsRpvQbdEC4a0ew__&Key-PairId=APKAJLOHF5GGSLRBV4ZA/.

[63] Gray JP, Müller VI, Eickhoff SB, Fox PT. Multimodal abnormalities of brain structure and function in major depressive disorder: a meta-analysis of neuroimaging studies. *American Journal of Psychiatry* [internet]. 2020 May 1 [cited 2021 Sept 15];177(5):422-434. Available from: https://www.ncbi.nlm.nih.gov/pmc/articles/PMC7294300/.

[64] Peña CJ, Nestler EJ. Progress in epigenetics of depression. *Progress in Molecular Biology and Translation*. [internet]. 2018;157:41-66. Available from: https://www.ncbi.nlm.nih.gov/pmc/articles/PMC6047749/.

[65] Kollert L, Schiele MA, Thiel C, Menke A, Deckert J, Domschke K. DNA hypomethylation of the Krüppel-like factor 11 (KLF11) gene promoter: a putative biomarker of depression comorbidity in panic disorder and of non-anxious depression? *Journal of Neural Transmission* [internet]. 2020 Nov [cited 2021 Sept 15];127(11):1539-1546. Available from: https://www.ncbi.nlm.nih.gov/pmc/articles/PMC7578153/.

[66] Saavedra K, Molina-Márquez AM, Saavedra N, Zambrano T, Salazar LA. Epigenetic modifications of major depressive disorder. *International Journal of Molecular Sciences* [internet]. 2016 Aug 5 [cited 2021 Sept 15];17(8):1279. Available from: https://www.ncbi.nlm.nih.gov/pmc/articles/PMC5000676/

[67] Misztak P, Pańczyszyn-Trzewik P, Nowak G, Sowa-Kućma M. Epigenetic marks and their relationship with BDNF in the brain of suicide victims. *PLoS ONE*

[internet]. 2020 [cited 2021 Sept 15]; 15(9): e0239335. Available from: https://storage.googleapis.com/plos-corpus-prod/10.1371/journal.pone.023933 5/1/pone.0239335.pdf?X-Goog-Algorithm=G OOG4-RSA-SHA256&X-Goog-Credential=wombat-sa%40plos-prod.iam.gserviceaccount.com%2F20211102%2 Fauto%2Fstorage%2Fgoog4_request&X-Goog-Date=20211102T193212Z&X-Goog-Expires=86400&X-Goog-SignedHeaders=host&X-GoogSignature=41419 237fb5a3ec236e574b72197fcd91a81d2914b0374d72536a949f6afbff725d8e5edff 90790c51c16bb7e76e9a664f10b90faf4b2a5dc6e6abf97096388edc8c1dc031f041e e8cdfec074c1d8da22c9fadc35b1808148e8e6d98049a8b746148ead444cd04c1386 c6aaae7b9ea3a1602eecd4498655484256b8503b45a590a65306a2cf2df2b9b96673 ca60cd4edc5cabbb7d47a0fdbb3d44465e1a9b2330a3848dc3167fb61aad81cdbb00e 2d0b25a615980251e654a8d388fd21ecae44250dd1145711c7acfd72665de9c9e8b4 c2dc3447c23b9c4d5cecb10c6e1eb94afa1019218294f2563e5e43ed48ebc7a89139 c1e55a1de24895d84c65a4d037b7b/.

[68] Ciuculete DM, Voisin S, Kular L, Welihinda N, Jonsson J, Jagodic M, Mwinyi J, Schiöth HB. Longitudinal DNA methylation changes at MET may alter HGF/c-MET signalling in adolescents at risk for depression. *Epigenetics* [internet]. 2020 Jun-Jul [cited 2021 Sept 20];15(6-7):646-663. Available from: https://www.nc bi.nlm.nih.gov/pmc/articles/PMC7574381/.

[69] Davies MN, Krause L, Bell JT, Gao F, Ward KJ, Wu H, Lu H, Liu Y, Tsai PC, Collier DA, Murphy T, Dempster E, Mill J; UK Brain Expression Consortium, Battle A, Mostafavi S, Zhu X, Henders A, Byrne E, Wray NR, Martin NG, Spector TD, Wang J. Hypermethylation in the ZBTB20 gene is associated with major depressive disorder. *Genome Biology*. [internet]. 2014 Apr 2 [cited 2021 Sept 20];15(4):R56. Available from: https://www.ncbi.nlm.nih.gov/pmc/articles/PMC 4072999/.

[70] Bernstein HG, Steiner J, Guest PC, Dobrowolny H, Bogerts B. Glial cells as key players in schizophrenia pathology: recent insights and concepts of therapy. *Schizophrenia Research*. 2015 Jan [cited 2021 Sept 20];161(1):4-18. Available from: https://www.researchgate.net/profile/Paul-Guest-2/publication/306012635 _Bernstein_Schizophrenia_Research_Glial_cells_in_schizophrenia/links/57aa0f4 e08ae42ba52ac0993/Bernstein-Schizophrenia-Research-Glial-cells-in-schizophr enia.pdf/.

[71] Goldman-Rakic PS, Selemon LD. Functional and anatomical aspects of prefrontal pathology in schizophrenia. *Schizophrenia Bull*etin [internet]. 1997 [cited 2021 Sept 20];23(3):437-58. Available from: https://academic.oup.com/schizophreniabu l letin/article/23/3/437/1886149/.

[72] Ju P, Cui D. The involvement of N-methyl-D-aspartate receptor (NMDAR) subunit NR1 in the pathophysiology of schizophrenia. *Acta Biochimica et Biophysica Sinica* [internet]. 2016 Mar [cited 2021 Sept 20];48(3):209-19. Available from: https://www.ncbi.nlm.nih.gov/pmc/articles/PMC4885128/.

[73] Reddy RD, Yao JK. Free radical pathology in schizophrenia: a review. *Prostaglandins, Leukototrienes & Essential Fatty Acids* [internet]. 1996 Aug [cited 2021 Sept 24];55(1-2):33-43. Available from: https://www.plefa.com/article/S095 2-3278(96)90143-X/pdf./.

[74] Osimo EF, Beck K, Reis Marques T, Howes OD. Synaptic loss in schizophrenia: a meta-analysis and systematic review of synaptic protein and mRNA measures. *Molecular Psychiatry* [internet]. 2019 Apr [cited 2021 Sept 24];24(4):549-561. Available from: https://www.ncbi.nlm.nih.gov/pmc/articles/PMC6004314/

[75] Ermakov EA, Dmitrieva EM, Parshukova DA, Kazantseva DV, Vasilieva AR, Smirnova LP. Oxidative stress-related mechanisms in schizophrenia pathogenesis and new treatment perspectives. *Oxidative Medicine and Cellular Longevity*. [internet]. 2021 Jan 23 [cited 2021 Sept 24];2021:8881770. Available from: https://www.ncbi.nlm.nih.gov/pmc/articles/PMC7847339/.

[76] Hany M, Rehman B, Azhar Y, et al. Schizophrenia. [Updated 2021 May 29]. In: *StatPearls* [ebook]. Treasure Island (FL): StatPearls Publishing; 2021 Jan. Available from: https://www.ncbi.nlm.nih.gov/books/NBK539864/#_NBK539864_pubdet_/ [cited 2021 Sept 24].

[77] Çöpoğlu ÜS, Igci M, Bozgeyik E, Kokaçya MH, İğci YZ, Dokuyucu R, Ari M, Savaş HA. DNA Methylation of BDNF Gene in schizophrenia. *Medical Science Monitor*. [internet]. 2016 Feb 6 [cited 2021 Sept 24];22:397-402. Available from: https://www.ncbi.nlm.nih.gov/pmc/articles/PMC4749043/.

[78] Khavari B, Cairns MJ. Epigenomic Dysregulation in schizophrenia: in search of disease etiology and biomarkers. *Cells* [internet]. 2020 Aug 5 [cited 2021 Sept 24];9(8):1837. Available from: https://www.ncbi.nlm.nih.gov/pmc/articles/PMC7463953/.

[79] Cariaga-Martinez A, Alelú-Paz R. Rethinking the epigenetic framework to unravel the molecular pathology of schizophrenia. *International Journal of Molecular Sciences*. [internet]. 2017 Apr 7 [cited 2021 Sept 24];18(4):790. Available from: https://www.ncbi.nlm.nih.gov/pmc/articles/PMC5412374/.

[80] Price AJ, Jaffe AE, Weinberger DR. Cortical cellular diversity and development in schizophrenia. *Molecular Psychiatry* [internet]. 2021 Jan [cited 2021 Sept 24];26(1):203-217. Available from: https://www.ncbi.nlm.nih.gov/pmc/articles/PMC7666011/.

[81] Gavin DP, Sharma RP. Histone modifications, DNA methylation, and schizophrenia. *Neuroscience & Biobehavioral Review*. [internet]. 2010 May [cited 2021 Sept 24];34(6):882-8. Available from: https://www.ncbi.nlm.nih.gov/pmc/articles/PMC2848916/.

[82] Pecorelli A, Cordone V, Schiavone ML, Caffarelli C, Cervellati C, Cerbone G, Gonnelli S, Hayek J, Valacchi G. Altered bone status in Rett syndrome. *Life* [internet]. 2021 Jun 3 [cited 2021 Sept 24];11(6):521. Available from: https://www.ncbi.nlm.nih.gov/pmc/articles/PMC8230033/.

[83] Ramirez JM, Karlen-Amarante M, Wang JJ, Bush NE, Carroll MS, Weese-Mayer DE, Huff A. The pathophysiology of Rett syndrome with a focus on breathing dysfunctions. *Physiology* [internet]. 2020 Nov 1 [cited 2021 Sept 24];35(6):375-390. Available from: https://journals.physiology.org/doi/abs/10.1152/physiol.00008.2020?rfr_dat=cr_pub++0pubmed&url_ver=Z39.882003&rfr_id=ori%3Arid%3Acrossref.org/.

[84] Lotan M, Ben-Zeev B. Rett syndrome. A review with emphasis on clinical characteristics and intervention. *Scientific World Journal* [internet]. 2006 Dec 6

[cited 2021 Sept 24];6:1517-41. Available from: https://www.ncbi.nlm.nih.gov/pmc/articles/PMC5917152/.

[85] Lotan M, Merrick J, Kandel I, Morad M. Aging in persons with Rett syndrome: an updated review. *Scientific World Journal* [internet]. 2010 May 4 [cited 2021 Sept 24];10:778-87. Available from: https://www.ncbi.nlm.nih.gov/pmc/articles/PMC5763738/.

[86] Tarquinio DC, Hou W, Neul JL, Berkmen GK, Drummond J, Aronoff E, Harris J, Lane JB, Kaufmann WE, Motil KJ, Glaze DG, Skinner SA, Percy AK. The course of awake breathing disturbances across the lifespan in Rett syndrome. *Brain & Development*. [internet]. 2018 Aug [cited 2021 Sept 24];40(7):515-529. Available from: https://www.ncbi.nlm.nih.gov/pmc/articles/PMC6026556/.

[87] Motil KJ, Lane JB, Barrish JO, Annese F, Geerts S, McNair L, Skinner SA, Neul JL, Glaze DG, Percy AK. Biliary tract disease in girls and young women with Rett syndrome. *Journal of Pediatric Gastroenterology*. [internet]. 2019 Jun;68(6):799-805. Available from: https://www.ncbi.nlm.nih.gov/pmc/articles/PMC6534452/.

[88] Horiuchi M, Smith L, Maezawa I, Jin LW. CX3CR1 ablation ameliorates motor and respiratory dysfunctions and improves survival of a Rett syndrome mouse model. *Brain, Behavior, and Immunity*. [internet]. 2017 Feb [cited 2021 Sept 24];60:106-116. Available from: https://www.ncbi.nlm.nih.gov/pmc/articles/PMC5531048/.

[89] Singh J, Lanzarini E, Santosh P. Autonomic dysfunction and sudden death in patients with Rett syndrome: a systematic review. *Journal of Psychiatry & Neuroscience*. [internet]. 2020 May 1 [cited 2021 Sept 24];45(3):150-181. Available from: https://www.ncbi.nlm.nih.gov/pmc/articles/PMC7828978/.

[90] Thurman AJ, Hoyos Alvarez C. Language performance in preschool-aged boys with nonsyndromic autism spectrum disorder or fragile X syndrome. *Journal of Autism and Developmental Disorders*. [internet]. 2020 May [cited 2021 Sept 30];50(5):1621-1638. Available from: https://www.ncbi.nlm.nih.gov/pmc/articles/PMC6699941/.

[91] Thurman AJ, McDuffie A, Hagerman R, Abbeduto L. Psychiatric symptoms in boys with fragile X syndrome: a comparison with nonsyndromic autism spectrum disorder. *Research in Developmental Disabilities*. [internet]. 2014 May [cited 2021 Sept 30];35(5):1072-86. Available from: https://www.ncbi.nlm.nih.gov/pmc/articles/PMC4009990/.

[92] Baker EK, Arpone M, Aliaga SM, Bretherton L, Kraan CM, Bui M, Slater HR, Ling L, Francis D, Hunter MF, Elliott J, Rogers C, Field M, Cohen J, Cornish K, Santa Maria L, Faundes V, Curotto B, Morales P, Trigo C, Salas I, Alliende AM, Amor DJ, Godler DE. Incomplete silencing of full mutation alleles in males with fragile X syndrome is associated with autistic features. *Molecular Autism*. [internet]. 2019 May 3 [cited 2021 Sept 30];10:21. Available from: https://www.ncbi.nlm.nih.gov/pmc/articles/PMC6499941/.

[93] Jin P, Warren ST. Understanding the molecular basis of fragile X syndrome. *Human Molecular Genetics*. [internet]. 2000 Apr 12 [cited 2021 Sept 30];9(6):901-8. Available from: https://academic.oup.com/hmg/article/9/6/901/618655/.

[94] Brasa S, Mueller A, Jacquemont S, Hahne F, Rozenberg I, Peters T, He Y, McCormack C, Gasparini F, Chibout SD, Grenet O, Moggs J, Gomez-Mancilla B, Terranova R. Reciprocal changes in DNA methylation and hydroxymethylation and a broad repressive epigenetic switch characterize FMR1 transcriptional silencing in fragile X syndrome. *Clinical Epigenetics*. [internet]. 2016 Feb 5 [cited 2021 Sept 30];8:15. Available from: https://www.ncbi.nlm.nih.gov/pmc/articles/PMC4743126/.

[95] Hagerman RJ, Berry-Kravis E, Hazlett HC, Bailey DB Jr, Moine H, Kooy RF, Tassone F, Gantois I, Sonenberg N, Mandel JL, Hagerman PJ. Fragile X syndrome. *Nature Reviews Disease Primers* [internet]. 2017 Sep 29 [cited 2021 Sept 30];3:17065. Available from: https://www.nature.com/articles/nrdp201765/.

[96] Nobile V, Pucci C, Chiurazzi P, Neri G, Tabolacci E. DNA methylation, mechanisms of *FMR1* inactivation and therapeutic perspectives for fragile X syndrome. *Biomolecules* [internet]. 2021 Feb 16 [cited 2021 Sept 30];11(2):296. Available from: https://www.ncbi.nlm.nih.gov/pmc/articles/PMC7920310/.

[97] McCullagh EA, Rotschafer SE, Auerbach BD, Klug A, Kaczmarek LK, Cramer KS, Kulesza RJ Jr, Razak KA, Lovelace JW, Lu Y, Koch U, Wang Y. Mechanisms underlying auditory processing deficits in Fragile X syndrome. *FASEB J.* [internet]. 2020 Mar [cited 2021 Sept 30];34(3):3501-3518. Available from: https://www.ncbi.nlm.nih.gov/pmc/articles/PMC7347277/.

[98] Razak KA, Dominick KC, Erickson CA. Developmental studies in fragile X syndrome. *Journal of Neurodevelopmental Disorders*. [internet]. 2020 May 2 [cited 2021 Sept 30];12(1):13. Available from: https://www.ncbi.nlm.nih.gov/pmc/articles/PMC7196229/.

[99] Engineer CT, Centanni TM, Im KW, Rahebi KC, Buell EP, Kilgard MP. Degraded speech sound processing in a rat model of fragile X syndrome. *Brain Research*. [internet]. 2014 May 20 [cited 2021 Sept 30];1564:72-84. Available from: https://www.ncbi.nlm.nih.gov/pmc/articles/PMC4034469/.

[100] Salcedo-Arellano MJ, Dufour B, McLennan Y, Martinez-Cerdeno V, Hagerman R. Fragile X syndrome and associated disorders: clinical aspects and pathology. *Neurobiology of Disease*. [internet]. 2020 Mar [cited 2021 Sept 30];136:104740. Available from: https://www.ncbi.nlm.nih.gov/pmc/articles/PMC7027994/.

[101] Razak KA, Dominick KC, Erickson CA. Developmental studies in fragile X syndrome. *Journal of Neurodevelopmental Disorders*. [internet]. 2020 May 2 [cited 2021 Sept 30];12(1):13. Available from: https://www.ncbi.nlm.nih.gov/pmc/articles/PMC7196229/.

[102] Banerjee A, Ifrim MF, Valdez AN, Raj N, Bassell GJ. Aberrant RNA translation in fragile X syndrome: from FMRP mechanisms to emerging therapeutic strategies. *Brain Research*. [internet]. 2018 Aug 15 [cited 2021 Sept 30];1693(Pt A):24-36. Available from: https://www.ncbi.nlm.nih.gov/pmc/articles/PMC7377270/.

[103] McLennan Y, Polussa J, Tassone F, Hagerman R. Fragile x syndrome. *Current Genomics* [internet]. 2011 May [cited 2021 Sept 30];12(3):216-24. Available from: https://www.ncbi.nlm.nih.gov/pmc/articles/PMC3137006/.

[104] Penagarikano O, Mulle JG, Warren ST. The pathophysiology of fragile x syndrome. *Annual Review of Genomics and Human Genetics*. [internet]. 2007

[cited 2021 Oct 2];8:109-29. Available from: https://www.annualreviews.org/doi/10.1146/annurev.genom.8.080706.092249?url_ver=Z39.88-2003&rfr_id=ori%3Arid%3Acrossref.org&rfr_dat=cr_pub++0pubmed/.

[105] Klusek J, Roberts JE, Losh M. Cardiac autonomic regulation in autism and Fragile X syndrome: a review. *Psychological Bulletin* [internet]. 2015 Jan [cited 2021 Oct 2];141(1):141-75. Available from: https://www.ncbi.nlm.nih.gov/pmc/articles/PMC4293203/.

[106] Roberts JE, Tonnsen B, Robinson A, Shinkareva SV. Heart activity and autistic behavior in infants and toddlers with fragile X syndrome. *American Journal on Intellectual and Developmental Disabilities.* [internet]. 2012 Mar [cited 2021 Oct 2];117(2):90-102. Available from: https://www.ncbi.nlm.nih.gov/pmc/articles/PMC3987776/.

[107] Sherman S, Pletcher BA, Driscoll DA. Fragile X syndrome: diagnostic and carrier testing. *Genetics in Medicine.* [internet]. 2005 Oct [cited 2021 Oct 2];7(8):584-7. Available from: https://www.ncbi.nlm.nih.gov/pmc/articles/PMC3110946/.

[108] Mishra S, Agarwalla SK, Potpalle DR, Dash NN. Rubinstein-Taybi syndrome with agenesis of corpus callosum. *Journal of Pediatric Neurosciences.* [internet]. 2015 Apr-Jun [cited 2021 Oct 2];10(2):175-7. Available from: https://www.ncbi.nlm.nih.gov/pmc/articles/PMC4489069/.

[109] Kumar P, Thota PN. Barrett's esophagus in Rubinstein-Taybi syndrome. *Cureus* [internet]. 2020 Nov 25 [cited 2021 Oct 2];12(11):e11709. Available from: https://www.ncbi.nlm.nih.gov/pmc/articles/PMC7769793/.

[110] Tatara Y, Kawakami N, Tsuji T, Miyasaka K, Ohara T, Nohara A. Rubinstein-Taybi syndrome with scoliosis. *Scoliosis* [internet]. 2011 Sep 30 [cited 2021 Oct 2];6:21. Available from: https://www.ncbi.nlm.nih.gov/pmc/articles/PMC3198739/.

[111] Wu Y, Xia Y, Li P, Qu HQ, Liu Y, Yang Y, Lin J, Zheng M, Tian L, Wu Z, Huang S, Qin X, Zhou X, Chen S, Liu Y, Wang Y, Li X, Zeng H, Hakonarson H, Zhuang J. Role of the ADCY9 gene in cardiac abnormalities of the Rubinstein-Taybi syndrome. *Orphanet Journal of Rare Diseases.* [internet]. 2020 Apr 22 [cited 2021 Oct 2];15(1):101. Available from: https://www.ncbi.nlm.nih.gov/pmc/articles/PMC7178576/.

[112] Schorry EK, Keddache M, Lanphear N, Rubinstein JH, Srodulski S, Fletcher D, Blough-Pfau RI, Grabowski GA. Genotype-phenotype correlations in Rubinstein-Taybi syndrome. *American Journal of Medical Genetics.* [internet]. 2008 Oct 1 [cited 2021 Oct 2];146A(19):2512-9. Available from: https://onlinelibrary.wiley.com/doi/10.1002/ajmg.a.32424/.

[113] Hennekam RC. Rubinstein-Taybi syndrome. *European Journal of Human Genetics.* [internet]. 2006 Sep [cited 2021 Oct 2];14(9):981-5. Available from: https://www.nature.com/articles/5201594/.

[114] Münevveroglu AP, Akgöl BB. Rubinstein-taybi syndrome: a case report. *Case Reports in Dentistry.* [internet]. 2012 [cited 2021 Oct 2];2012:483867. Available from: https://www.ncbi.nlm.nih.gov/pmc/articles/PMC3443573/.

[115] DaCosta J, Brookes J. Infantile glaucoma in Rubinstein-Taybi syndrome. *Eye* [internet]. 2012 Sep [cited 2021 Oct 2];26(9):1270-1. Available from: https://www.ncbi.nlm.nih.gov/pmc/articles/PMC3443829/.

[116] Spena S, Gervasini C, Milani D. Ultra-rare syndromes: the example of Rubinstein-Taybi syndrome. *Journal of Pediatric Genetics*. [internet]. 2015 Sep [cited 2021 Oct 2];4(3):177-86. Available from: https://www.ncbi.nlm.nih.gov/pmc/articles/PMC4918723/.

[117] Milani D, Manzoni FM, Pezzani L, Ajmone P, Gervasini C, Menni F, Esposito S. Rubinstein-Taybi syndrome: clinical features, genetic basis, diagnosis, and management. *Italian Journal of Pediatrics*. [internet]. 2015 Jan 20 [cited 2021 Oct 2];41:4. Available from: https://www.ncbi.nlm.nih.gov/pmc/articles/PMC4308897/.

[118] IA Qureshi, MF Mehler. 2018. Epigenetic mechanisms underlying nervous system diseases. - *Handbook of Clinical Neurology, 147:* 43-45. doi: 10.1016/B978-0-444-63233-3.00005-1.

[119] JCI Susan, J Harrison, CL Paul, M Frommer High sensitivity mapping of methylated cytosines - *Nucleic Acids Research* [internet] 1994 Available from: https://academic.oup.com/nar/article-abstract/22/15/2990/1087317.

Chapter 7

Therapies for Parkinson's Disease: Mechanisms and Current Trends

Amrutha K[1] and Sarika Singh[2,*]

[1]Academy of Scientific & Innovative Research (AcSIR), Ghaziabad, India
[2]Department of Neuroscience and Ageing Biology,
Division of Toxicology and Experimental Medicine,
CSIR-Central Drug Research Institute, Lucknow, India

Abstract

Parkinson's disease (PD) is one of the most common neurodegenerative disorders due to the loss of dopaminergic neurons of the substantia nigra pars compacta (SNpc). The neuronal loss in the brain leads to motor and non-motor indications which in later stages aggravate with cognitive decline. Treatment options available to date only provide symptomatic relief by focusing on the restoration of dopamine in the brain and could not prevent the disease progression, suggesting the need of novel interventions that can solve the suffering and improve the quality of life of the patient. Research studies and technology development has suggested new dimensions to be targeted in search of a novel therapeutic alternative for PD patients. Among those, stem cell therapy is one that opens up a new window in treatment in which the progenitor cells are grafted into patients to regenerate dopaminergic neurons in the brain. Advancement in the neurosurgical procedures also offers the same, like deep brain stimulation (DBS) being used to treat the advanced stages of PD and brings hope in the future of PD treatment. This chapter discusses different therapeutic approaches that influence the quality of life of PD patients.

---

* Corresponding Author's Email: sarika_singh@cdri.res.in.

In: New Perspectives in Neuroscience
Editors: Prachi Srivastava, Neha Srivastava and Prekshi Garg
ISBN: 978-1-68507-754-9

Introduction

Parkinson's disease (PD) is one of the most common neurodegenerative disorders which is characterised by motor symptoms including bradykinesia, resting tremor, rigidity and postural instability (Tarakad et al., 2017). Several non-motor symptoms like hyposmia, REM sleep behaviour disorder, depression, and constipation precede the motor symptoms of PD (Tarakad et al., 2017). Sporadic PD that occurs randomly in a population is the most common form of PD. However, genetic defects can also be a reason for PD pathogenesis, which include mutations in genes like SNCA, LRRK2 (leucine-rich repeat kinase 2), Parkin, PINK1, and DJ-1. Mutation in SNCA gene results in the aggregation of α-synuclein to form lewy bodies, a well-known pathological hallmark in PD pathology (Borsche et al., 2020). A long-term exposure to pesticides like rotenone, paraquat and organophosphates, dysregulated iron metabolism, infection (post-encephalitic PD) and drugs (antipsychotics) can be secondary causes of PD (Singh et al., 2007, Goldman, S. M., 2014). In regard to PD diagnosis, only clinical symptoms and scoring procedures are available and investigations are on-going to search for peripheral diagnostic marker for PD. The degeneration of the dopaminergic nigrostriatal pathway results in the reduction of dopamine level, a neurotransmitter which sends messages between nerve cells to regulate the motor activities (Segura-Aguilar et al., 2014). During physiological conditions if the dopamine content is in excess in the cytosol then it is degraded by the two enzymes monoamine oxidase (MAO-B) and catechol *ortho*-methyltransferase (COMT) (Segura-Aguilar et al., 2014). However, under pathological conditions, the decreased level of dopamine further reduced by the action of these two enzymes and worsen the conditions. As a therapeutic option the dopamine supply to body was considered. However, this was not a successful strategy as dopamine could not cross the blood brain barrier therefore, the precursor of dopamine i.e., levodopa is administrated along with carbidopa, inhibitor of dopa decarboxylase enzyme therefore prevent the conversion of levodopa to dopamine in periphery and facilitate the increased level of levodopa in brain. Once levodopa enters the brain, it is converted into dopamine by dopa decarboxylaseenzyme. The peripheral decarboxylase enzyme may also break down levodopa before reaching the brain results in the lesser availability of dopamine in the brain (Calne, D. B., 1993) and such degradation could be lessened by carbidopa. Anticholinergic drugs like trihexyphenidyl and benztropine is also used for PD treatment that can block the acetylcholine production and reduce the muscle stiffness. Amantadine is another drug that has some similar effects in PD patients (Calne, D. B., 1993). Ergot derivatives like bromocriptine and pergolide are dopamine receptor agonists that act on D1 and D2 receptors and increase the receptor activity (Calne, D. B., 1993). Selegiline and rasagiline are inhibitors of MAO-B whereas drugs like entacapone, tolcapone are COMT inhibitors that can protect the dopamine from metabolism inside the brain (Calne, D. B., 1993, Singh et al., 2007). These agents are still less effective and are inadequate to subside the disease totally and in-depth investigations and repurposing may be one of the quick strategies for research and development. Such repurposing strategy may involve the molecule having interference in any of the neuropathological mechanisms of PD pathogenesis. Recent study shows that in experimental PD model, the metformin, a well-known hypoglycaemic agent, exerts its cytoprotective effects by activating nuclear factor erythroid 2-related factor 2 (Nrf2)/heme-oxygenase (HO)-1 pathway, which in turn, is dependent on AKT activation and it also upregulates PGC-1α that helps in mitochondrial biogenesis and reduce the ROS levels (Katila et al., 2021) which can be a pronounced drug of choice for PD. Drug repurposing have been preferred as a choice for PD treatment and clinical trials are continuing in this area (Table 1).

Table 1. Repurposing of drugs in the clinical trial for Parkinson's disease

Drugs	Clinical outcomes	Number of patients	Reference
Zuranolone	Adjunct therapy has improved tremor, motor and non-motor experiences in PD patients.	14	Bullock et al., 2021
Multi-strain probiotic (Hexbio)	Improved bowel opening frequency and whole gut transit time in PD patients with constipation.	55	Ibrahim et al., 2020
Nilotinib	Shows stable UPDRS scores over 27 months	63	Pagan et al., 2021
Pioglitazone	Lower incidence of PD among diabetic patient	8396	Brakedal et al., 2017
Febuxostat and inosine combination	Significantly improved MDS-UPDRS Part III scores	29	Watanabe et al., 2020
Lovastatin	Decreasing motor symptom progression and slowing the dopaminergic neuronal decline measured by ^{18}F-dopa PET	77	Lin et al., 2021
Glycopyrrolate	Significant reduction in the severity of PD-related sialorrhea	28	Mestre et al., 2020

Abbreviations: MDS-UPDRS, Movement Disorder Society-Unified Parkinson's Disease Rating Scale; PET, Positron Emission Tomography.

Therapies Targeting Intracellular Mechanism

Oxidative Stress

Neurons are postmitotic and high energy requiring cells which is fulfilled by mitochondria via process called oxidative phosphorylation. The movement of electrons through different protein complexes from complex I to complex IV promotes a proton gradient between mitochondrial membrane and matrix which will generate a potential difference that helps in the production of ATP (Puspita et al., 2017). Reactive Oxygen Species (ROS) is generated inside the mitochondria during this process preferably when complex I and complex III protein becomes leaky and has been regulated by different antioxidative mechanisms involving glutathione (GSH) and superoxide dismutase (SOD) (Dorszewska et al., 2021). If such generated ROS like hydroxyl radical, peroxides, superoxide accumulates it causes the oxidative stress capable to damage the cell through initiating various degenerating events.

Table 2. Antioxidants under research for treatment of Parkinson's disease

Drugs	Mechanism involved	References
Caffeic acid	Metabolic and mitochondrial alterations observed in fibroblasts from PD patients	Deus et al., 2021
Curcumin	Pre-treatment helps in improving maximal respiration and ATP associated respiration in paraquat induced model of PD	Abrahams et al., 2021
Coreopsis lanceolate flower extract	Inhibits H2O2-induced ROS generation and caspase-3 activation in PC12 Cells	Kim et al., 2021
Polyphenols	Inhibits neuroinflammation	Singh et al., 2020
Hydroxytyrosol and oleuropein aglycone	Increased survival of C. elegans after heat stress, improved locomotive behaviour	Brunetti et al., 2020

During physiological conditions such generated ROS could be neutralized with cellular antioxidants like GSH, which remains in abundance in mitochondrion however, the dysfunctional mitochondrion is the major cause of oxidative stress and one of the neurodegenerative mechanism in PD pathology (Puspita et al., 2017). Both ROS and Reactive Nitrogen Species (RNS) have been accumulated in the dopaminergic neurons. RNS includes nitroxyl anion, nitrosonium cation, higher oxides of nitrogen, S-nitrosothiols, and dinitrosyl iron complexes derived from nitric oxide (NO). The NOS (nitric oxide synthase) catalysed reaction of L-arginine produce NO intracellularly in neurons which acts as messengers in CNS (Nathan et al., 1994). The NO react with ROS and generate the peroxynitrite that promote nitration and later produce the hydroxyl radicals (Tipton et al., 1993) and jointly these free radicals induce the oxidative stress in neurons. In view of considerable role of oxidative stress in PD pathology various antioxidants have been suggested to be used in PD therapeutics (Table 2).

Protein Aggregation

Lewy bodies are the pathological hallmark of PD pathology and suggested the role of protein clearance mechanism in PD pathology. Lewy bodies consist of filamentous material, α-synuclein which is translated from SNCA gene. The α-synuclein form oligomers that interact with the membrane phospholipids and disrupt the membrane and makes the synaptic vesicles leaky. The interaction of α-synuclein with dopamine interferes in the release of dopamine from the nerve ending and also renders the dopaminergic neurons more sensitive for cytotoxicity and collectively contributes to the PD pathology. Cellular protein homeostasis is maintained through regular synthesis of proteins and degradation of misfolded/unfolded proteins utilizing protein clearance mechanism. The ubiquitin-proteasome system (UPS) is one of the considerable protein clearance mechanism in PD pathology as recently we have reported the depleted proteasome activity in PD pathology. UPS essentially require the tagging of ubiquitin through three enzymes involving ubiquitin activating enzyme (E1), ubiquitin conjugating enzymes (E2) and ubiquitin ligases (E3)a process called polyubiquitination. This process gives the protein a specific identity to be recognised by the 26S proteasome for degradation. The depleted tagging of ubiquitin to target protein or depleted UPS will cause the accumulation of misfolded/unfolded proteins and cause protein aggregation. The evidence from the post mortem brain of PD patient reveals that SKp1 protein, a component of E3 ubiquitin ligases levels have been reduced considerably in SNpc region suggesting its pathological role.

The preclinical studies are now going on restricting the propagation of α-synuclein by developing antibodies using passive and active immunisation (Fields et al., 2019). Anti-sense oligonucleotide and ribonucleic acid (RNA) interference techniques are also under consideration for disrupting α-synuclein synthesis (Sapru et al., 2006, McCormack et al., 2010). In a recent study, CRISPR tool is used to enhance the transcription factor EB (TFEB) and metalloprotease 17 (ADAM17) genes in HEK293T cell lines. These genes are meant for lysosomal biogenesis and have secretase activity to cleave the insoluble proteins respectively thus to decrease the protein aggregation (Siddiqui et al., 2021). In the cells, α-synuclein oligomerization and conformation were measured by fluorescence resonance energy transfer (FRET) with fluorescent α-synuclein biosensors which gives a hope for the early detection of the mistranslated protein (Braun et al., 2021). Prasinezumab or PRX002, a monoclonal antibody that is undergoing phase II clinical trial has reduced the serum α-synuclein by 97% in the phase I clinical trial by targeting the C-terminus of aggregated α-synuclein (Schenk et al., 2017, Jankovic et al., 2018). Another antibody BIIB054 (Biogen) that targets the N-terminal portion of α-synuclein reduces the propagation of α-synuclein pathology improves the motor implications in mice model of PD (Weihofen et al., 2019). Another approach was to design the α-synuclein fragments or α-synuclein-mimicking epitopes (AFFITOPE PD01A) to induce the immune response and these are in phase II clinical trial (Fields et al., 2019).

Neurotransmitter Targeting

Deficiency in the neurotransmitter systems in the brain other than dopamine also experienced the clinical symptoms of PD. Safinamide, selective, reversible monoamine oxidase-B inhibitor which has both dopaminergic and non-dopaminergic (glutamatergic) properties. In the EU, safinamide is approved for the treatment of mid to late stage PD patients as an add-on therapy with a stable dose of levodopa (Caccia et al., 2006). A recent study proved that the nanoparticles with multiple enzymatic activities purified from ground water can enhance the synaptic transmission by increasing neurotransmitter production and activating the nicotinic acetylcholine receptors (nAChRs), activate the antioxidant enzyme system, and increase the number of mitochondria and ribosomes in cells (Guo et al., 2021). The cholinesterase inhibitors, rivastigmine and donepezil are clinically being used for Alzheimer's disease and been tested for the improvement of gait in PD patients. Observation suggested the positive implications of both in gait improvement (Henderson et al., 2016). Clinical trials are now being conducted on noradrenaline reuptake inhibitors, methylphenidate and atomoxetine to assess whether these drugs have any satisfactory effect on gait, balance and motor function (NCT02879136) and results yet to be declare.

Inflammation

The neuroinflammatory responses are also one of the neurodegenerative events in PD pathology as reviewed previously (Joshi and Singh, 2018). The immune responses in the CNS are primarily initiated by the microglia and are crucial for the proper regulation of homeostasis and tissue structures. If the inflammation persists due to the failure in the termination mechanism or due to increased stimuli like secreted signalling factors from the neurons, then the condition will be complicated and chronic. Reports have suggested the critical role of neuroinflammatory responses in PD pathology (Hirsch et al., 2012; Joshi and Singh, 2018) and PET quantification done in PD brain also affirm the hypothesis, as prominent microglial activation was observed (Bartels et al., 2010).

Studies suggested that NLRP3 inhibitor, MCC950 suppressed the microglial inflammasome activation, improved the neuronal physiology and reduces the α-synuclein aggregation in PD model (Gordon et al., 2018) suggesting a new approach for development of novel therapeutic target for PD. Agents utilised for preclinical trials includes 7-nitroindazole (improves striatal dopamine depletions) (Yokoyama et al., 2008), Minocycline, NSAIDS (anti-inflammatory action), Pioglitazone (Reduction of dopaminergic cell dead and microgliosis) (Pajares et al., 2020) have showed the anti-inflammatory and neuroprotective activity. Semaglutide, a glucagon-like peptide 1 (GLP1) synthetic analogue is also in phase II clinical trial due to its neuroprotective and anti-inflammatory activity (NCT03659682). Kv1.3, a voltage-gated potassium channel, upregulated in response to α-synuclein aggregation and has an ability to augment the neuroinflammation. A recent study demonstrated that Kv1.3-specific small-molecule inhibitor PAP-1(5-(4-phenoxy butoxy) psoralen significantly inhibited the neuroinflammation and neurodegeneration in experimental animal model of PD (Sarkar et al., 2020).

Therapies Promoting Neuronal Regeneration via Stem Cell

Regeneration therapy for the replacement of the lost dopaminergic neurons became the area of interest nowadays. A study demonstrated the differentiation of mesenchymal stem cell (MSC) into dopaminergic neurons and its settlement in SNpc regionby the stimulation of electromagnetic field (EMF) in rat model. MSCs that were exposed to EMF with 400 μT increase the BDNF in brain and subsequently lead to increased tyrosine hydroxylase neurons in SNpc (Jadidi et al., 2016). This proposes the impact of stem cell therapy in PD. A recent study was based on excavating the mechanism behind the action of adipose-derived human mesenchymal stem cell which can protects the dopaminergic neurons and it was found that pentraxin 3 is the key factor involved in it. Pentraxin 3 is a human mesenchymal stem cell secreted protein. The experiment using human recombinant pentraxin 3 treatment on PD mice prevented the apoptosis, neuronal degeneration and increased neuronal terminals in SNpc and striatum that proved the same (Lian et al., 2021). A clinical trial has been initiated by the physician of Kyoto University Hospital in partnership with Center for iPS Cell Research and Application on dopaminergic progenitors generated from induced pluripotent stem cells (iPSCs). In this trial, seven patients have received the bilateral grafts of allogenic iPSC-derived cells (https://www.cira.kyoto-u.ac.jp/e/research/find ing.html). An embryonic stem cell derived neural precursor cells are under clinical trial now to assess its efficacy on Parkinson's Disease (NCT03119636). Gene therapy techniques are also under phase I clinical trial to increase the dopamine level in the striatum by manipulating two genes tyrosine hydroxylase (TH) and aromatic L-amino acid decarboxylase (AADC) which are crucial for the dopamine production. An adeno-associated virus therapy which carry AADC gene is introduced into the putamen of PD patient who are in advanced stage of disease. The preliminary results suggested an increased enzyme activity in the brain regions (Christine et al., 2019) and further studies are on-going.

Deep Brain Stimulation (DBS)

DBS has been used and being well established for solving the motor features of PD. Electrodes have been implanted inside the brain to stimulate the sub thalamic nucleus (STN) and globus pallidus internus (GPi) through surgical procedure. It is preferably used when the available treatment regime is not sufficient for the improvement of quality of life of a patient. DBS has several adverse effects too. An open label trial using DBS is beneficial for PD patients by improved tremor score in their early days after diagnosis (Grabli et al., 2013). The pedunculopontine nucleus has been trialled as a new target in DBS for gait problems (Stefani et al., 2007). A transcutaneous magnetic spinal cord stimulation (SCS) study has also been done to demonstrate its safety and efficacy on freezing the gait in PD patients and the results proved that the SCS is safe, improved the gait and UPDRS-III score by 17% (Menezes et al., 2020).

Conclusion

The drug interventions available in the market are not enough to reverse the progression of PD. The number of patients suffering from the disease is still increasing due to the increasing geriatric population. Extensive research is on-going in this problem to rescue the patient from the disease pathology. Therapies not only for curing the disease condition but also measures for prevention are under consideration like antioxidants, PD vaccines etc. A greater understanding of the disease pathway is crucial for finding out the perfect solution for it and the researchers had won in this scenario up to some extent and still the in-depth investigations in regard to multidimensional neurodegenerative signaling are required.

References

Abrahams, S., Miller, H. C., Lombard, C., van der Westhuizen, F. H. and Bardien, S., 2021. Curcumin pre-treatment may protect against mitochondrial damage in LRRK2-mutant Parkinson's disease and healthy control fibroblasts. *Biochemistry and Biophysics Reports,* 27, p. 101035.

Bartels, A. L., Willemsen, A. T. M., Doorduin, J., De Vries, E. F. J., Dierckx, R. A. and Leenders, K. L., 2010. (11C)-PK11195 PET: quantification of neuroinflammation and a monitor of anti-inflammatory treatment in Parkinson's disease? *Parkinsonism & related disorders,* 16(1), pp. 57-59.

Borsche, M., Pereira, S. L., Klein, C., Grünewald, A. Mitochondria and Parkinson's Disease: Clinical, Molecular, and Translational Aspects. *Journal of Parkinson's Disease*, (Preprint), 2020, 1-16.

Brakedal, B., Flones, I., Reiter, S. F., Torkildsen, O., Dolle, C., Assmus, J., Haugarvoll, K., Tzoulis, C. Glitazone use associated with reduced risk of Parkinson's disease. *Mov. Disord.* 2017, 32, 1594-1599.

Braun, A. R., Liao, E. E., Horvath, M., Kalra, P., Acosta, K., Young, M. C., Kochen, N. N., Lo, C. H., Brown, R., Evans, M. D. and Pomerantz, W. C., 2021. Potent inhibitors of toxic alpha-synuclein identified via cellular time-resolved FRET biosensors. *npj Parkinson's Disease,* 7(1), pp. 1-17.

Brunetti, G., Di Rosa, G., Scuto, M., Leri, M., Stefani, M., Schmitz-Linneweber, C., Calabrese, V. and Saul, N., 2020. Healthspan Maintenance and Prevention of Parkinson's-like Phenotypes with Hydroxytyrosol and Oleuropein Aglycone in C. elegans. *International journal of molecular sciences,* 21(7), p. 2588.

Bullock, A., Kaul, I., Li, S., Silber, C., Doherty, J. and Kanes, S. J., 2021. Zuranolone as an oral adjunct to treatment of Parkinsonian tremor: A phase 2, open-label study. *Journal of the Neurological Sciences*, 421, p. 117277.

Caccia, C., Maj, R., Calabresi, M., Maestroni, S., Faravelli, L., Curatolo, L., Salvati, P. and Fariello, R. G., 2006. Safinamide: from molecular targets to a new anti-Parkinson drug. *Neurology,* 67(7 suppl 2), pp. S18-S23.

Calne, D. B., 1993. Treatment of Parkinson's disease. *New England Journal of Medicine*, 329(14), pp. 1021-1027.

Christine, C. W., Bankiewicz, K. S., van Laar, A. D., et al., Magnetic resonance imaging-guided phase 1 trial of putaminal AADC gene therapy for Parkinson's disease. *Ann Neurol.* 2019; 85(5): 704-14.

Cyranoski, D. Trials of embryonic stem cells to launch in China. *Nature.* 2017; 546(7656): 15-6.

Deus, C. M., Pereira, S. P., Cunha-Oliveira, T., Teixeira, J., Simões, R. F., Cagide, F., Benfeito, S., Borges, F., Raimundo, N. and Oliveira, P. J., 2021. A mitochondria-targeted caffeic acid derivative reverts cellular and mitochondrial defects in human skin fibroblasts from male sporadic Parkinson's disease patients. *Redox Biology*, p. 102037.

Dorszewska, J., Kowalska, M., Prendecki, M., Piekut, T., Kozłowska, J. and Kozubski, W., 2021. Oxidative stress factors in Parkinson's disease. *Neural Regeneration Research*, 16(7), p. 1383.

Fields, C. R., Bengoa-Vergniory, N. and Wade-Martins, R., 2019. Targeting Alpha-Synuclein as a Therapy for Parkinson's Disease. *Front Mol Neurosci.;* 12: 299.

Goldman, S. M., 2014. Environmental toxins and Parkinson's disease. *Annual review of pharmacology and toxicology*, 54, pp. 141-164.

Gordon, R., Albornoz, E. A., Christie, D. C., Langley, M. R., Kumar, V., Mantovani, S., Robertson, A. A. B., Butler, M. S., Rowe, D. B., O'Neill, L. A., et al., Inflammasome inhibition prevents alpha-synuclein pathology and dopaminergic neurodegeneration in mice. *Sci. Transl. Med.* 2018, 10.

Grabli, D., Karachi, C., Folgoas, E., et al., Gait disorders in parkinsonian monkeys with pedunculopontine nucleus lesions: A tale of two systems. *J Neurosci.* 2013; 33(29): 11986-93.

Guo, S., Feng, R., Hao, W., Sun, S., Wei, C. and Hu, X., 2021. Nanoparticles with Multiple Enzymatic Activities Purified from Groundwater Efficiently Cross the Blood-Brain Barrier, Improve Memory, and Provide Neuroprotection. *ACS Applied Bio Materials*, *4* (7), pp. 5503-5519.

Henderson, E. J., Lord, S. R., Brodie, M. A., Gaunt, D. M., Lawrence, A. D., Close, J. C., Whone, A. L. and Ben-Shlomo, Y., 2016. Rivastigmine for gait stability in patients with Parkinson's disease (ReSPonD): a randomised, double-blind, placebo-controlled, phase 2 trial. *The Lancet Neurology,* 15(3), pp. 249-258.

Hirsch, E. C., Vyas, S. and Hunot, S., 2012. Neuroinflammation in Parkinson's disease. *Parkinsonism & related disorders,* 18, pp. S210-S212.

Ibrahim, A., Ali, R. A. R., Manaf, M. R. A., Ahmad, N., Tajurruddin, F. W., Qin, W. Z., Desa, S. H. M. and Ibrahim, N. M., 2020. Multi-strain probiotics (Hexbio) containing MCP BCMC strains improved constipation and gut motility in Parkinson's disease: A randomised controlled trial. *Plos one*, 15(12), p. e0244680.

Jadidi, M., Biat, S. M., Sameni, H. R., Safari, M., Vafaei, A. A. and Ghahari, L., 2016. Mesenchymal stem cells that located in the electromagnetic fields improves rat model of Parkinson's disease. *Iranian journal of basic medical sciences,* 19(7), p. 741.

Jankovic, J., Goodman, I., Safirstein, B., et al., Safety and Tolerability of Multiple Ascending Doses of PRX002/RG7935, an Anti-α-Synuclein Monoclonal Antibody, in Patients With Parkinson Disease: A Randomized Clinical Trial. *JAMA Neurol.* 2018; 75(10): 1206-14.

Joshi, N. and Singh, S., 2018. Updates on immunity and inflammation in Parkinson disease pathology. *Journal of neuroscience research*, 96(3), pp. 379-390.

Katila, N., Bhurtel, S., Park, P. H. and Choi, D. Y., 2021. Metformin attenuates rotenone-induced oxidative stress and mitochondrial damage via the AKT/Nrf2 pathway. *Neurochemistry International,* p. 105120.

Kim, H. D., Lee, J. Y., Park, J. Y., Kim, D. H., Kang, M. H., Seong, H. A., Seo, K. H. and Ji, Y. J., 2021. Neuroprotective Effects of Coreopsis lanceolata Flower Extract against Oxidative Stress-Induced Apoptosis in Neuronal Cells and Mice. *Antioxidants,* 10(6), p. 951.

Lian, C., Huang, Q., Zhong, X., He, Z., Liu, B., Zeng, H., Xu, N., Yang, Z., Liao, C., Fu, Z. and Guo, H., 2021. Pentraxin 3 secreted by human adipose-derived stem cells promotes dopaminergic neuron repair in Parkinson's disease via the inhibition of apoptosis. *The FASEB Journal,* 35(7), p. e21748.

Lin, C. H., Chang, C. H., Tai, C. H., Cheng, M. F., Chen, Y. C., Chao, Y. T., Huang, T. L., Yen, R. F. and Wu, R. M., 2021. A Double-Blind, Randomized, Controlled Trial of Lovastatin in Early-Stage Parkinson's Disease. *Movement Disorders,* 36(5), pp. 1229-1237.

McCormack, A. L., Mak, S. K., Henderson, J. M., et al., Alpha-synuclein suppression by targeted small interfering RNA in the primate substantia nigra. *PLoS One.* 2010; 5(8): e12122.

Menezes, J. R., Carra, R. B., Nunes, G. A., da Silva Simões, J., Teixeira, M. J., Duarte, K. P., de Andrade, D. C., Barbosa, E. R., Marcolin, M. A. and Cury, R. G., 2020. Transcutaneous magnetic spinal cord stimulation for freezing of gait in Parkinson's disease. *Journal of Clinical Neuroscience,* 81, pp. 306-309.

Mestre, T. A., Freitas, E., Basndwah, A., Lopez, M. R., de Oliveira, L. M., Al-Shorafat, D. M., Zhang, T., Lui, J. P., Grimes, D. and Fox, S. H., 2020. Glycopyrrolate Improves Disability From Sialorrhea in Parkinson's Disease: A 12-Week Controlled Trial. *Movement Disorders,* 35(12), pp. 2319-2323.

Nathan, C., Xie, Q. W. (1994) Nitric oxide synthases: roles, tolls, and controls. *Cell* 78:915-918.

Pagan, F. L., Wilmarth, B., Torres-Yaghi, Y., Hebron, M. L., Mulki, S., Ferrante, D., Matar, S., Ahn, J. and Moussa, C., 2021. Long-Term Safety and Clinical Effects of Nilotinib in Parkinson's Disease. *Movement Disorders,* 36(3), pp. 740-749.

Pajares, M., I Rojo, A., Manda, G., Boscá, L. and Cuadrado, A., 2020. Inflammation in Parkinson's disease: mechanisms and therapeutic implications. *Cells,* 9(7), p. 1687.

Puspita, L., Chung, S. Y. and Shim, J. W., 2017. Oxidative stress and cellular pathologies in Parkinson's disease. *Molecular brain*, 10(1), pp. 1-12.

Sapru, M. K., Yates, J. W., Hogan, S., et al., 2006. Silencing of human alpha-synuclein in vitro and in rat brain using lentiviral-mediated RNAi. *Exp Neurol.* 198(2): 382-90.

Sarkar, S., Nguyen, H. M., Malovic, E., Luo, J., Langley, M., Palanisamy, B. N., Singh, N., Manne, S., Neal, M., Gabrielle, M. and Abdalla, A., 2020. Kv1. 3 modulates neuroinflammation and neurodegeneration in Parkinson's disease. *The Journal of clinical investigation*, 130(8), pp. 4195-4212.

Schenk, D. B., Koller, M., Ness, D. K., et al., First-in-human assessment of PRX002, an anti-α-synuclein monoclonal antibody, in healthy volunteers. *Mov Disord.* 2017; 32(2): 211-8.

Segura-Aguilar, J., Paris, I., Muñoz, P., Ferrari, E., Zecca, L. and Zucca, F. A., 2014. Protective and toxic roles of dopamine in Parkinson's disease. *Journal of Neurochemistry*, 129(6), pp. 898-915.

Siddiqui, A. N., 2021. *Activating TFEB and ADAM17 using CRISPRa to treat neurodegenerative diseases.* [online] Available from: http://lup.lu b.lu.se/student-papers/record/9060855/.

Singh, N., Pillay, V. and Choonara, Y. E., 2007. Advances in the treatment of Parkinson's disease. *Progress in neurobiology*, 81(1), pp. 29-44.

Singh, S. S., Rai, S. N., Birla, H., Zahra, W., Rathore, A. S. and Singh, S. P., 2020. NF-κB-mediated neuroinflammation in Parkinson's disease and potential therapeutic effect of polyphenols. *Neurotoxicity Research,* 37(3), pp. 491-507.

Stefani, A., Lozano, A. M., Peppe, A., et al., Bilateral deep brain stimulation of the pedunculopontine and subthalamic nuclei in severe Parkinson's disease. *Brain.* 2007; 130(Pt 6): 1596-607.

Tarakad, A. and Jankovic, J., 2017, April. Diagnosis and management of Parkinson's disease. In *Seminars in neurology* (Vol. 37, No. 02, pp. 118-126). Thieme Medical Publishers.

Tipton, K. F., Singer, T. P. (1993) Advances in our understanding of the mechanisms of the neurotoxicity of MPTP and related compounds. *J Neurochem* 61:1191-1206.

Watanabe, H., Hattori, T., Kume, A., Misu, K., Ito, T., Koike, Y., Johnson, T. A., Kamitsuji, S., Kamatani, N. and Sobue, G., 2020. Improved Parkinsons disease motor score in a single-arm open-label trial of febuxostat and inosine. *Medicine,* 99(35).

Weihofen, A., Liu, Y., Arndt, J. W., et al., Development of an aggregate-selective, human-derived α-synuclein antibody BIIB054 that ameliorates disease phenotypes in Parkinson's disease models. *Neurobiol Dis.* 2019; 124: 276-88.

Yokoyama, H., Takagi, S., Watanabe, Y., Kato, H. and Araki, T., 2008. Role of reactive nitrogen and reactive oxygen species against MPTP neurotoxicity in mice. *Journal of neural transmission,* 115(6), pp. 831-842.

Chapter 8

Mitophagy, Autophagy and Angiogenesis - The Collaborative Partners of Alzheimer's Disease

Shivanjali Saxena[1,2,*] **and Sushmita Jha**[1]
[1]Indian Institute of Technology Jodhpur, Jodhpur, India
[2]Institute of Systems Genetics, NYU Langone Health, New York, New York, USA

Abstract

Neurodegeneration is a process of losing the structure and/or functionality of neurons and their death causing inefficiency in the working of the brain. It's an umbrella term for the pathology of various diseases such as Parkinson's disease (PD), Amyotrophic lateral sclerosis (ALS) and Alzheimer's disease (AD). Although increasing age is the most common factor for developing AD or PD, there are several causes that remain unexplored. Genetic and environmental factors also contribute to the etiology of these diseases but the mechanism of their contribution to the initiation of these diseases is a topic of debate. For Alzheimer's disease, beta-amyloid plaques are the primary pathological lesion but mechanisms behind the formation of these plaques need to be elucidated. Genetic polymorphism, brain inflammation, cerebral hypoperfusion and heredity are suggested as potential mechanisms behind the onset of this disease. In 1991, Blass and Gibson proposed mitochondrial dysfunction and disrupted neuronal metabolisms as the early features of AD. After that, a lot of studies have documented the dysfunctional mitochondria in the AD affected neurons due to impaired mitophagy. Dysfunctional mitochondria widely enhance the ROS

* Corresponding Author's Email:saxena.1@iitj.ac.in.

In: New Perspectives in Neuroscience
Editors: Prachi Srivastava, Neha Srivastava and Prekshi Garg
ISBN: 978-1-68507-754-9

production that exacerbates mitochondrial damage further leading to aberrant processing of amyloid precursor proteins and pTau proteins causing amyloid beta plaques and neurofibrillary tangles. Recently it was also proposed that AD is mediated by pathological angiogenesis. Post-mortem studies have also revealed enhanced angiogenesis in the hippocampus, midfrontal cortex, substantia nigra pars compacta, and locus coeruleus of AD brains as compared to normal brains. Risk factors such as hypertension, smoking, apolipoprotein E (APOPE), etc. are common for both cardiovascular diseases and AD suggesting a link between the two. Pathological angiogenesis in the AD brain can be caused as a result of inflammation and oligaemia due to vascular injury and cerebral perfusion respectively. This results in the deposition of amyloid Beta plaques and secretion of a neurotoxic peptide that kill neurons worsening the disease. The objective of this chapter is to explore the relation between mitophagy and angiogenesis in the pathology of Alzheimer's disease. Exploring this will help in the development of new and more effective interventions for treating pathology as well as cognitive impairments related to AD and other neurodegenerative diseases.

Keywords: Alzheimer's disease, neurodegeneration, autophagy, mitophagy, angiogenesis, inflammation

Introduction

Nervous system is an essential system for an efficient working of human body. It plays a critical role in perceiving our surroundings through sensory neurons and performing motor as well as vital functions through motor neurons. This implies that effective working of neurons is very important for our survival. Loss of structure, function or both of neurons results in a very devastating class of diseases termed as "Neurodegenerative diseases." Neurodegenerative diseases consist of Alzheimer's diseases (AD), Parkinson's disease (PD) and Amyotrophic lateral sclerosis (ALS) (Vissers, Ming, and Song 2019). Neurodegeneration causes inefficiency in the working of the brain thereby leading to problems in the functioning of day-to-day routine work. These diseases have become very common due to increased life expectancy as ageing is considered the most common cause for them. According to 2017 report on Alzheimer's disease around 5.5 million Americans are suffering from this disease. By mid-century this number is proposed to grow to 13.8 million. Dynamics of this disease indicates that a new case generates every 66 seconds that will decrease to 33seconds by the year 2050. These estimates make this diseases one of the most common diseases in the coming years (Association 2017).

In 1907, AD was firstly reported but it got recognition as the most common cause of dementia and death after 70 years (Katzman 1976, Wilson et al. 2012). Dementia is a syndrome with number of causes and its symptoms consists of difficulties with memory, language and cognitive skills. These symptoms occur when neurons are damaged in the areas related to these activities. This is why AD is ultimately fatal because after a point of time nerve damage occurs in areas related to bodily functions such as swallowing, walking etc (Barker et al. 2002). In 1960 invention of electron microscopy resulted into getting new insights about ultra-structural changes underlying lesions (senile plaques and neurofibrillary tangles) related to AD (Selkoe 2001). During 1970s the neurochemical cause behind dementing symptom of AD was discovered. It was observed in AD patients that acetylcholine producing neurons were undergoing severe damage resulting in the dementing symptoms of AD. Till date the FDA approved drugs for AD are based on the inhibitors of acetylcholine degradative enzymes acetyl transferase and acetylcholinesterase. It is implied that inhibiting these degradative enzymes will help in enhancing levels of acetylcholine in the synaptic cleft. In the early 1980s it came to knowledge that in AD various neurotransmitter systems are altered thereby decreasing the efficiency of acetylcholine-based drugs. The advancement of symptoms from mild to severe varies from person to person depending on the degradation rate of neurons. Diagnosis of AD is not a single step process. It requires comprehensive medical examination by physicians and neurologists. Dementia can be identified but deciding on the cause of dementia is a time taking process.

Pathology of Alzheimer's Disease

In an adult healthy brain there are about 100 billion neurons and around 100 trillion synapses that are formed by the axon terminals and dendrites of the neurons (Association 2017). Synapses allow information to travel rapidly through the neuronal circuit. This creates the cellular basis of sensations, movements, memories, emotions, thoughts and skills. Pathology of AD is characterized with the accumulation of fibrous protein known as "Beta-amyloid Plaques" (Aβ Plaques) (Villemagne et al. 2013). Outside the neuron, fragmented protein amyloid beta gets accumulated while inside neurons there is accumulation of abnormal form of Tau protein termed as Tau tangles (Bateman et al. 2012). These plaques were initially observed in the post-mortem of AD brains. This led to a long-term debate that these pathological features can be tombstone of the disease and not the initiators. Pathology of AD can be divided into three phases: Biochemical, Cellular and Clinical. In the biochemical phase, Amyloid beta plaques and tau tangles contribute to the pathology of AD by interfering with neuronal communication at the synapses and blocking nutrient and other essential molecules transport within the cell respectively, thereby causing cell death. They exert "proteopathic" stress not only on neurons but also on other cells such as microglial and endothelial cells. They also interacts with Aβ and Tau and disrupt their normal functionality (Palop and Mucke 2010). Temporal sequence of these disruptions is undefined but the age-related deficiencies mark the hallmark of AD. Age related deficiency in the proteostatic network of cell results in accumulation of protein aggregates which in turn disturbs molecular network of protein folding (Labbadia and Morimoto 2015). The lysosomal/endolysosomal system, specifically autophagy and mitophagy are key regulators of protein aggregates. Dysfunction of autophagy and mitophagy causes accretion of Amyloid beta plaques and tau tangles (Nixon 2013, Fang et al. 2019, Kerr et al. 2017). Contribution of autophagy and mitophagy will be further discussed in the chapter. Initial response effects of proteopathy are reversible as brain cells deal with this for long time through maintenance of homeostasis in the proteostatic network and through synaptic plasticity mechanisms (Labbadia and Morimoto 2015). This is the critical point when stresses of biochemical phase lead to cellular phase of AD. Inflammatory pathways play an important role in maintaining homeostasis but when they turn into chronic and irreversible pathological process, the disease progression becomes inexorable. This state is the clinical phase of AD where cellular network is no longer able to maintain the cellular homeostasis (De Strooper and Karran 2016).

As discussed above, pathology of AD is directed through various mechanisms or various cell specific effects of the same mechanism. Amyloid beta plaques and tau tangles interact with proteins and receptors of cellular populations in the brain, in a cell-specific manner and exert multiple or same effects on the functionality of cells. For instance, Amyloid beta plaques interact with receptor for advanced glycation end products (RAGE) on neurons thereby causing oxidative stress while interacting with RAGE on microglial enhances its inflammatory response. In case of endothelial cells, it leads to reverse transport of Amyloid beta across the blood brain barrier (Deane et al. 2012). Dramatic inflammation in brain and brain shrinkage together with lot of debris has been observed in the brains of the advanced AD patients (Association 2017). Neuroinflammation plays a critical role in the pathophysiology of AD. Interaction between neurons and microglia are evident through transcriptomic and epigenomic studies (Mathys et al. 2019). These studies reveal down-regulation of neuronal functions while innate immune response is up-regulated in the brains of AD patients.

Effective CNS functioning is a result of regulated transport across the blood brain barrier (BBB) and optimum coupling between cerebral blood flow (CBF) and neuronal activity (Benarroch 2007). Optimal Performance of these two critical functions require the synchronized activity of neurovascular unit of brain. This neurovascular unit consists of endothelial cells, perivascular neurons, astrocytes and vascular smooth muscle cells (VSMC) (Benarroch 2007). Role of neurovascular unit in pathology of AD has been discussed in various studies.

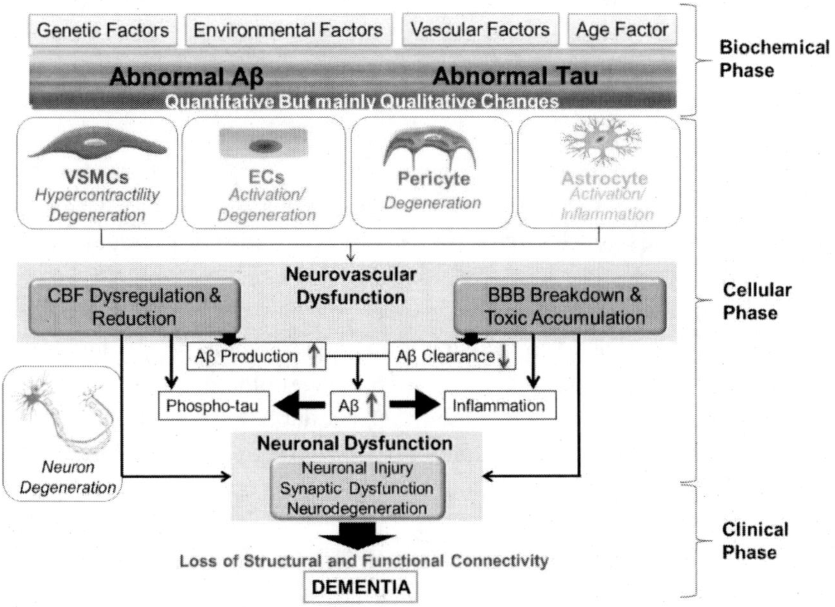

Figure 1. Pathology of Alzheimer's disease. Phases of Alzheimer's disease consisting of cellular changes, neurovascular and neuronal dysfunction are shown. These pathological hallmarks are responsible for symptoms such as dementia of Alzheimer's disease.

Neurovascular Unit Functioning in Normal Brain

The functioning between regional CBF and neuronal activity is termed as functional hyperemia which is elicited by enhanced synaptic activity. Enhanced energy consumption by astrocytes and active neurons leads to high metabolic signal that contributes to hyperemia (Iadecola 2004, Koehler, Gebremedhin, and Harder 2006). Activity associated upsurge in CBF is caused by release of several vasodilators such as extracellular potassium (K^+) and hydrogen ions (H^+), adenosine, nitric oxide (NO)s, prostanoids and neurotransmitters (Koehler, Gebremedhin, and Harder 2006, Iadecola 2004, Filosa et al. 2006). These vasodilators are released by endothelial cells, perivascular neurons and astrocytes. Glutamate released from active excitatory synapses is not a vasodilator, but it induces the release of various vasodilators such as NO and prostanoids. Perivascular astrocytes are important player in neurovascular coupling that occurs as a result of excitatory synaptic activity (Benarroch 2007). Contact between pericytes of capillaries or smooth muscle cells of parenchymal arterioles and astrocytic end foot is essential for signalling mechanism caused by synaptic activity. Excitatory synaptic activity causes release of glutamate that stimulates metabotropic glutamate receptors in astrocytes. This causes release of intracellular Ca^{+2} signal through astrocytic end feet towards the astrocytic network. This enhanced level of Ca^{+2} leads to release of several signals such as K^+, derivative of arachidonic acid and NO (Rossi 2006, Filosa et al. 2006, Iadecola 2004). These factors elicit relaxation response of smooth muscle in parenchymal arterioles. Increase in perivascular K^+ leads to activation of inward rectifying K^+ channels present in smooth muscle cells in arterioles. This results in vasodilation and cell hyper-polarization (Koehler, Gebremedhin, and Harder 2006). Neurons are also known to play role in regulation of CBF through synthesis of various neuropeptides such as Neuropeptide Y (NPY) and Calcinonin gene related peptide (CGRP) (Suzuki et al. 1989). Vasoactive neuropeptides secreted by brainstem cholinergic neurons, cortical GABAergic interneurons and monoaminergic neurons are send through processes that ends onto cerebral micro-vessels and astrocytes thereby regulating local CBF (Iadecola 2004, Hamel 2006). Along with neurons, pericytes that are present on the exterior side of the basement membrane of the capillary endothelium also regulate local CBF. They also contribute towards maintenance of vascular integrity, vascular remodeling and angiogenesis (Zlokovic 2005).

The neurovascular unit efficiently regulates chemical composition of neuronal microenvironment not only through maintenance of local CBF but also through maintaining molecular transfer across BBB. The structural integrity of BBB is due to presence of tight junctions between capillary endothelial cells but astrocytes are majorly responsible for its maintenance and functionality (Abbott, Rönnbäck, and Hansson 2006). BBB is an extremely metabolic unit that consists of specialized transport systems present at its luminal (blood-facing) as well as abluminal (brain-facing) sides. Function of luminal side transporter is to carry nutrients such as glucose, nucleosides and amino acids towards the brain whereas abluminal side transporters perform function of elimination of toxic substances that includes metabolic waste products, excitatory neurotransmitters and amyloid β peptides (Deane, Wu, and Zlokovic 2004, Zlokovic 2005). BBB also performs the function of maintaining pool of amyloid β peptides in brain as compared to plasma and cerebral spinal fluid (CSF) which in normal conditions is in equilibrium. Interaction of soluble amyloid β peptides with RAGE regulates its influx while low density lipoprotein receptor present on endothelium regulates its efflux across the brain. Apolipoproteins (apo) E and J are known to regulate metabolism and clearance of amyloid β peptides (Zlokovic 2005, Deane, Wu, and Zlokovic 2004).

Dysfunction of Neurovascular Unit in Alzheimer's Disease

Experimental evidences suggest that neurovascular unit dysfunction leads to aberrant changes in cerebrovascular structure in AD which is one of the hallmarks of AD's pathology (Iadecola 2004). Here we will discuss the mechanism of neurovascular unit dysfunction and vascular dysfunction and their effects in AD. PET and SPECT analysis of AD patient's brain shows reduction of glucose metabolism and oxygen utilization (Kisler et al. 2017). Most pronounced pathological regions in AD brains have least glucose metabolism (Friedland et al. 1985). As discussed above BBB transporters play major role in maintenance of environment across BBB. A severe deficit of glucose transporters has been observed in AD brain as compared to normal aged-match control brains (Haxby et al. 1988). The site of glucose transporter production in brain is capillary endothelium which is damaged in AD thereby causing deficiency in glucose transporters (Deutsch and Tweedy 1987). Due to disruption of neurovascular unit, lowered cerebral blood flow is observed in AD brains as compared to normal aged brains. Association between lowered cerebral blood flow and reduced glucose and oxygen metabolism has also been observed in AD brains (Deutsch and Tweedy 1987).

Key pathological feature of AD i.e., accumulation of amyloid β peptides known as amyloid plaques is followed by its accumulation in blood vessels termed as amyloid angiopathy (Zlokovic 2005). Studies suggest role of amyloid β peptides in the disruption of neurovascular unit components. Aβ is known to kill pericytes which in turn may accelerate neurovascular aberration (Park et al. 2014, Sagare et al. 2013, Wilhelmus et al. 2007). Even accumulation of low levels of soluble Aβ before their aggregation is sufficient enough to cause global vascular impairment. This was observed in APP Swedish mutation expressing mice (*Tg2576*) in which cerebrovascular reactivity to endothelium-dependent vasodilators was reduced while it was increased in response to vasoconstrictors that act on smooth muscle cells (Iadecola et al. 1999). Interaction of Aβ with RAGE in brain endothelium leads to generation of endothelin-1 (ET-1) that causes reduction of CBF in *Tg2576* mice (Deane et al. 2003, Deane et al. 2012). Aβ also induces NADPH-oxidase that leads to generation of reactive oxygen species (ROS) by cortical neurons further causing vascular dysfunction (Park et al. 2005). Aβ also binds to CD36 scavenger receptor and causes oxidative stress in cerebral blood vessel (Park et al. 2011). This leads to reduced neurovascular coupling in the AD brain. Oxidative stress also tampers NO-arbitrated vasodilation through production of superoxide ions (Girouard and Iadecola 2006). These superoxide ions produce peroxynitrite as a result of interaction with NO thereby reducing its accessibility for vasodilation (Iadecola 2004). Peroxynitrite further attenuates vasodilation through inhibition of vasodilator prostaglandins synthesis (Zlokovic 2005, Benarroch 2007). Transgenic mice models of AD depicted inability of VSMCs to clear Aβ in the walls of the vessels thereby causing cerebral amyloid angiopathy and compromised vascular reactivity (Bell et al. 2009, Kimbrough et al. 2015). Similar to AD patients, mice model of AD showed hypercontractile phenotype of VSMCs and weakened endothelium (dependent & independent) relaxation resulting in tempered CBF response (Chow et al. 2007). Additionally Aβ shows toxic effect on endothelial cells via disruption of tight junction proteins (occluding &claudin) expression and also through activation of local inflammatory response (Marco and Skaper 2006). Aβ has also shown to cause endothelial cell apoptosis as observed in AD transgenic mice model (Folin et al. 2006). Apolipoprotein-E (ApoE) has been observed to modulate cytotoxic effects of Aβ on endothelial cells in an in vitro model. One of the isoform of ApoE, ApoE-4 increases the toxic effects while another isoform ApoE-2 decreases the toxic effects of Aβ on endothelial cells (Folin et al. 2006).

These studies implies that Aβ imparts vasoactive and vasculotoxic effects on cerebral vasculature thereby affecting various neurovascular unit components that in turn cause CBF deregulation mediated effects. As discussed above neurovascular unit dysfunctions in AD leads multifactorial effects. Some of the mediators of these affects such as NO, apolipoprotein-E and Endothelin-1 are the known the players in the process of angiogenesis (Ziche et al. 1994, Wu et al. 2014, González-Pecchi et al. 2015). Therefore, further we will discuss about the contribution of angiogenesis towards the pathology of AD.

Angiogenesis and Alzheimer's Disease

Epidemiological studies data reveals that chances of getting an AD in high-risk population decreases significantly through the prolonged use of certain drugs. These drugs belong to the category of non-steroidal anti-inflammatory agents (NSAIDs), histamine H2-receptor blockers, lipid-lowering statins and calcium-channel blockers (In'T Veld et al. 2001, Forette et al. 1998, McGeer, Schulzer, and McGeer 1996). Initially neuroinflammation treatment was thought to be the cause of the protective effects of these drugs but not all of these drugs possess anti-inflammatory activity. Though, these preventive agents were found to be having inhibitory effect on angiogenesis and aberrant angiogenesis was observed to be the hallmark of AD pathology. This leads to need for exploring role of angiogenesis in AD together with other markers of AD pathology.

Association of vascular dysfunction with the dementia was reported in 1873, when unusual distorted vasculature in the brains of mentally disturbed patients was observed after their death (Tuke 1873). Further reports on abnormal vasculature were made in brains of several AD and dementia patients through autopsy (Bastai 1933, Campbell, Alexander, and Putnam 1938, Cerletti 1910). The characteristic traits of these abnormal micro vessels were kinky, torturous, looped and twisted vessels with numerous amounts of amyloid deposits on their walls (Hassler 1967, Ravens 1978, Beskow, Hassler, and Ottosson 1971, Tagliavini et al. 1990). The deformed vasculature was found to be more prominent in areas where plaques, tangles and reactive astrocytes are initially found and are most dense in the AD brains. These areas are hippocampus and temporoparietal regions of the brain (Tagliavini et al. 1990, Hassler 1967). In normal aged brains blood vessels show smooth and cylindrical profile with branching of capillaries and arterioles without any deformity on the surface (Scheibel, Duong, and Jacobs 1989, Scheibel, Wechsler, and Brazier 1986). Branching of blood vessels to form new blood vessels is termed as angiogenesis. Normal angiogenesis depicting arc, gentle loops or straight line like structures are observed in the normal aged brains. Envelope of perivascular neuronal plexus was also observed on these normal blood vessels (Scheibel, Duong, and Jacobs 1989, Scheibel, Wechsler, and Brazier 1986). Ultrastructure analysis of AD brains showed an entirely different picture as compared to normal aged brains. Cortical biopsies of AD brains depicted an aberrant angiogenesis marked by highly irregular contours of the capillaries studded with lots of knobs like structures (Scheibel, Duong, and Jacobs 1989, Scheibel, Wechsler, and Brazier 1986). Abnormal angiogenesis was marked by exaggeratedly thickened & torturous basement membrane with the absence of neuronal plexus (Mancardi et al. 1980, Kidd 1964, Miyakawa et al. 1986, Miyakawa and Kuramoto 1989, Miyakawa and Uehara 1979). Not just the vascular structure but also its components vary in AD brains as compared to normal aged brains. In normal brains, collagen provides support to basement membrane of capillaries but in case of AD brains it was observed to be spilling out or dissecting the membrane's layer of vessels (De la Torre and Mussivan 1993, Athanikar et al. 1988, Perlmutter et al. 1988). AD brains are also marked by presence of amyloid masses and damaged endothelial cells in capillaries spreading from blood vessel walls to adjacent parenchyma and also adjacent to narrowed lumens (Miyakawa et al. 1986, Higuchi et al. 1987).

Enhanced expression of angiogenesis factors such as vascular endothelial growth factor (VEGF), transforming growth factor β (TGF-β) and tumor necrosis factor α (TNFα) is also observed in aberrant vasculature and in intrathecal areas of AD brains (Tarkowski et al. 2002, Perlmutter et al. 1990). Reports suggest that VEGF co-localizes with Aβ Plaques in brains of AD patients (Yang et al. 2004). In vitro experiments also revealed that VEGF binds to Aβ Plaques with strong affinity resulting in its unavailability under hypoperfusion that may contribute to vascular dysfunction in AD brains (Yang et al. 2004). As discussed above ROS generated by Aβ Plaques leads to damage of brain endothelium. This causes generation of thromobogenic regions on the walls of vessels that result in intravascular aggregation of thrombin (Ciallella et al. 1999). Thrombin accumulation causes stimulation of angiogenesis and β-Amyloid precursor protein production in the endothelial cells. Thrombin mediated production of β-Amyloid precursor protein by endothelial cells occurs through receptor mediated protein kinase C pathway (Ciallella et al. 1999). Progressive deposition of this precursor protein causes accumulation of Aβ Plaques which further generates more ROS and thereby causes more endothelium damage (Vagnucci Jr and Li 2003). Other processes that stimulate angiogenesis in AD brains are: Hypoxia caused due to hypoperfusion that is known to occur in elderly brains is one of the potent inducers of angiogenesis. Hypoxia activates HIF-1α that mediates the transcription of various angiogenic and inflammatory factors thereby inducing angiogenesis and an inflammatory response (Kalaria et al. 1998); Inflammatory mediators such as Interleukin-6, monocyte chemoattractant protein-1 and TNF-α found in AD brain also stimulates angiogenesis (Grammas and Ovase 2001); The neurofibrillary tangles found in AD brains contains heparin sulphate proteoglycan that is a substrate for basic fibroblast growth factor (bFGF) and binds to it with great affinity thereby stimulating angiogenesis (Siedlak et al. 1991); Gene expression of Thrombospondin which is an endogenous angiogenesis inhibitor also decreases near lesions in the Alzheimer's brain. This leads to induction of proangiogenic environment in these sites (Buee et al. 1992).

It is evident through above discussed studies that angiogenesis is the one of the primary drivers of pathogenesis of AD. As preventive agents of AD show anti-angiogenic properties, it implies that anti-angiogenic interventions together with other measures can prove beneficial in the treatment of AD. As discussed above, proteostatic systems of cells in the brain of AD patients are disrupted. Due to which accumulation of protein aggregates occurs in AD brains. Autophagy and Mitophagy are two most common cellular systems for maintenance of proteosomal balance in the cell. Exploring co-relation between these proteostatic systems and angiogenesis will pave way for novel therapeutic interventions.

Autophagy and Mitophagy in Alzheimer's Disease

Protein homeostasis is important for healthy living of cell. This is maintained through tightly regulated synthesis of proteins or their degradation. Autophagy is an intracellular process in which cytosolic components of cells are degraded and recycled in lysosomes/vacuoles for maintenance of protein homeostasis (Klionsky et al. 2011). In mammalian cells, autophagy can be classified into three classes: Chaperone-mediated autophagy (CMA); micro-autophagy; macro-autophagy (Mizushima et al. 2008). CMA occurs in cytosolic proteins consisting of KFERQ motif (Cuervo 2010). Due to this motif, these proteins are selectively targeted for degradation in the lysosomal lumen (Cuervo 2010).

In micro-autophagy there is non-selective introduction of small quantities of cytoplasm into the lysosome for degradation. Macroautophagy is the primary type of autophagy and perform protein degradation on a large scale (He and Klionsky 2009). Autophagy in general refers to macroautophagy which is the largest contributor of autophagy process. The process of autophagy is mediated through phosphorylation events of Unc 51-like autophagy activating kinase 1 (ULK1) and AMP-activated protein kinase (AMPK) by mammalian target of rapamycin complex 1 (mTORC1) (He and Klionsky 2009). Inhibition of mTORC1 induces the process of autophagy through activation of autophagy related protein (Atg) complex that initiates autophagosome formation (Díaz-Troya et al. 2008). Autophagy starts with the formation of an "isolation membrane" from phagophore (small cup-shaped membrane precursor) or pre-autophagosomal structure (PAS). Isolation membrane seizes a region of cytoplasm that is to be degraded to form a double-membrane-limited autophagosome (Xie and Klionsky 2007, Axe et al. 2008). This is followed by fusion of lysosome or late endosome with an outer membrane of autophagosome thereby developing an autolysosome or an amphisome respectively. As lysosomes and endosomes consist of variety of hydrolases, degradation of sequestered materials is initiated in the autolysosomes and amphisomes. Vacuolar [H+] ATPase proton pump is required for acidification of autolysosomes. It is crucial for cathepsins activation for proteolysis of substrates inside autolysosomes. Once the process of substrate digestion is completed in autolysosomes, smaller and less dense lysosomes containing mainly lysosomal hydrolases are released. This completes the process of autophagy with the restoration of lysosomes in the cell.

Autophagy deregulation in AD can occur in three different stages of autophagy process: Autophagosome formation; lysosome mediated autophagosome clearance; autophagic flux. Autophagic flux is the dynamic equilibrium between rate of substrate sequestration and substrate degradation by the autophagosome (Wong and Cuervo 2010, Chu 2006). Uniquely extensive accumulation of autophagosme related vesicular structures (AVs) and dystrophic neurites has been observed in AD brains as compared to other age-related neurodegenerative brains. In AD brains, high number of dystrophic neuritis is present and AVs are unable to clear the cytoplasmic burden of these dystrophic neuritis (Nixon and Cataldo 2006). Also, number of AVs increases in normal neuritis present in AD brains. This implies an enormous burden of undigested proteins that leads to accumulation of non-native proteins in the AD brain. Lysosomal proteolysis is disrupted in neurons of AD brains that causes selective disruption of autophagy related axonal transport (Nixon 2013). This is the major reason of axonal dystrophy that occurs in AD brains and is characterized by AVs accumulation (Nixon and Yang 2011). Studies suggest that major cause of autophagy dysfunction in AD brain is disruption of proteolytic clearance ability of lysosomes (Nixon and Yang 2011). Electron-dense autolysosomes and autophagosomes consisting partially or undigested substrates are found in the AD brains (Cataldo et al. 1995, Nixon et al. 2005). These AVs accumulate in the neurons even though the expression of lysosomal hydrolases is very high (Cataldo et al. 1995, Cataldo et al. 1996). Abundant lysosomes present in the dystrophic neuritis fuse with these accumulated AVs. This type of pattern occurs when there is inhibition of lysosomal degradation due to deletion of one or more cathepsins, use of cysteine protease or lysosomal enzyme inhibitors. This implies that disruption of cathepsins, cysteine proteases or lysosomal enzymes can contribute towards the autophagy related pathology in AD brains (Papassotiropoulos et al. 2000, Koike et al. 2000, Ivy et al. 1984). Cytoplasmic adaptor Phosphatidylinositol binding clathrin assembly protein (PICALM) plays role in clathrin-mediated endocytosis and therefore is required in autophagy. In AD brains it's observed that PICALM is abnormally cleaved because of which levels of full-length protein is decreased (Wolfe et al. 2013, Lee et al. 2010). This leads to disruption of synthesis as well as maturation of autophagosomes. Autophagy is an important regulator of both production and degradation of Aβ (Ntsapi et al. 2018). Disruption of autophagososmes in AD brains not only result in its accumulation due to their inefficiency in degrading Aβ but also results in their additional accumulation (Kurtishi et al. 2019). AVs contain high amount of active enzymes (γ-Secretase complex) that are capable of producing Aβ (Ntsapi et al. 2018). Confirmatory to this, increase in the production of Aβ with the induction of autophagy has been observed (Nilsson et al. 2013). Autophagy is also responsible for tau clearance. Although ubiquitin protease system is responsible for tau degradation, studies suggest that accumulation of Tau increases when autophagy-lysosome system is dysfunctional (Di Meco et al. 2019, Uddin et al. 2018). In evidence of this, studies have shown that autophagy is directly related to phosphorylation of Tau (Piras et al. 2016). Hyperphosphorylation of Tau was observed in the autophagy-deficient mice suggesting that autophagy can be an alternative pathway for phosphorylated Tau degradation and clearance (Uddin et al. 2019, Inoue et al. 2012). Recent finding also reported that intracellular accumulation of Tau protein inhibits histone deacetylase-6 (HDAC6) activity thereby causing dysfunction of autophagy (Uddin et al. 2018). Along with autophagy, Aβ and Hyperphosphorylated Tau also regulate mitophagy in AD brains.

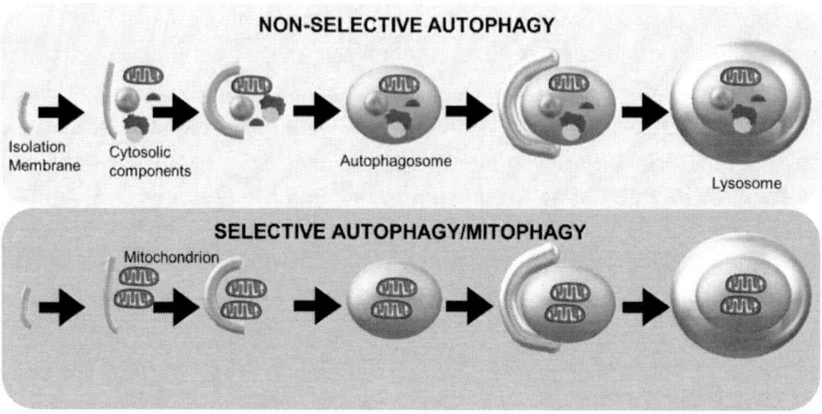

Figure 2. Mechanism of autophagy. Non-selective autophagy process for degradation of cellular components includes formation of autophagosome and lysosome. Selective autophagy degrades specific components of cell such as mitochondrion. Process of mitochondrion degradation is termed as mitophagy.

Mitophagy is the selective clearance of damaged mitochondria by autophagy (Fang 2019).Mitochondria are responsible for energy production and redox signalling of cell. It also promotes developmental and synaptic plasticity. In AD brains as well as in AD transgenic animal models, mitochondrial dysfunction together with accumulation of damaged mitochondria is observed (Reddy 2006). The major pathway for clearing damaged mitochondria and maintaining mitochondrial homeostasis is mitophagy. It is evident through studies that mitophagy is impaired in the brains of AD patients (Reddy and Oliver 2019). In transgenic APP mice, enhanced mRNA expression of mitochondrial energy metabolism genes is reported implying towards impairment of energy metabolism with AD progression (Reddy et al. 2004). This may be due to excessive production of free radicals by Aβ in mitochondria that leads to its damage. To compensate the energy metabolism of dysfunctional mitochondria, increase in mitochondrial encoded genes was observed in APP mice (Reddy et al. 2004). Interaction of Aβ and mitochondrial fission protein Drp1 is also reported that is responsible for mitochondrial fragmentation in AD brains (Manczak, Calkins, and Reddy 2011). Similar findings are also reported with phosphorylated Tau protein leading to excessive fragmentation of mitochondria (Manczak and Reddy 2012). In AD brains, Aβ and Tau proteins causes most damage to mitophagy through reduction of parkin and PINK1 proteins that are essential for successful mitophagy pathway (Oliver and Reddy 2019). This also causes enhanced hyperphosphorylation of Tau and synaptic dysfunction together with dysfunctional mitochondrial transport (Calkins et al. 2011). In a recent study it was found that there is an interaction between Aβ oligomers and autophagic vacuoles that results in axonal dysfunction and inhibition of axonal transport of mitochondria (Tammineni et al. 2017). These studies suggest that both autophagy and mitophagy are deregulated in AD by Aβ and Tau proteins through various mechanisms. We have discussed the aberrant angiogenesis in AD brains and its contribution to pathogenesis of AD. Role of Aβ and Tau proteins in context of angiogenesis in AD is also explored in this chapter. Autophagy, mitophagy and angiogenesis are three aspects of AD pathology therefore now we will discuss the correlation between the three. Exploring the possible contribution of these three aspects together in AD will help in getting further insight into the pathology of AD and will also help in understanding its cellular and molecular links as a complete system.

Relation between Autophagy/Mitophagy and Angiogenesis in Alzheimer's Disease

Autophagy and angiogenesis depict a very dynamic relation with each other. Reports suggest that deficiency in autophagy may be one of the mechanisms to cause dysfunction of endothelial cells (Park et al. 2017). Endothelial cell paracrine signalling depends upon secretion of angiogenic factors through release of exosomes (Hassanpour, Cheraghi, et al. 2018). Stimulation of autophagy promotes the biogenesis of exosomes in endothelial cells. These exosomes are seen to carry angiogenic factors such as von Willebrand factor (vWF) and vascular endothelial growth factor receptor2 (VEGFR2) (Torisu et al. 2013). In vascular injury, exocytosis is the first line of defense in endothelial cells. In this process Weibelpalade bodies which are specific secretory vessels within endothelial cells are formed and they contain active molecules such as vWF. Near or within the autophagosomes in endothelial cells these palade bodies are reported to be found. It has also been observed that inhibition of autophagy causes inhibition of vWF's in vitro secretion (Valentijn et al. 2011). There are studies which suggest that in diabetes impaired function of endothelial cells could be reversed through autophagy induction as autophagy improves angiogenic capacity of HUVECs exposed to high glucose (Fetterman et al. 2016).In case of esophageal cancer similar relation between autophagy and angiogenesis was observed. In the esophageal squamous cell carcinoma cell line, effect of autophagy inhibitor was tested in presence of radiotherapy. It was observed that autophagy inhibitor inhibited radiation induced autophagy thereby increasing radiosensitivity of the tumor. Also autophagy inhibition resulted in increase in apoptosis and decrease in cellular proliferation as well as angiogenesis (Chen et al. 2015). Hypoxia which is a prime regulator of angiogenesis was also found to regulate the autophagy through HIF-α mediated induction of *bnip3* and *bnip1* (BCL interacting protein). Which are BH3-only proapoptotic genes (Bellot et al. 2009). BNIP3, one of the target genes of HIF-1α is reported to inhibit its stabilization through BNIP3 dependent mitophagy. This leads to mitophagy dependent mitigation of tumor promoting activity, including angiogenesis in mammary tumor model (Chourasia and Macleod 2015). Studies also report that chronic hypoxia aggravates the pathology of AD through activation of AMPK that further inhibits mTOR signalling pathway that causes autophagy induction which further aggravates the disease due to its dysfunction (Liu et al. 2015). mTOR signalling pathway is known to modulate various angiogenic factors such as NO and angiopoietins (Karar and Maity 2011). Rampamycin, the known inhibitor of mTOR has shown positive effects on vascular system. It promotes endothelial cell functioning and enhances angiogenesis as well in animal models (Lin et al. 2013, Lesniewski et al. 2017). In AD, enhanced mTOR signalling is reported. This may be the cause of enhanced aberrant angiogenesis in AD brains. Although, In a study it was reported that Aβ inhibits the proliferation capacity of the human brain vascular endothelial cells and decrease angiogenesis through induction of self-digesting autophagy (Hayashi et al. 2009). But, in case of AD pathology as autophagy is dysfunctional, aberrant angiogenesis occurs. Aβ is known to stimulate both autophagy and angiogenesis in AD brains thereby proposing direct relation between the two. In AD, although Aβ induce autophagy but it is dysfunctional due to which it leads to accumulation of Aβ and aggravates the pathology of AD. Contradictory to above mentioned studies, there are several studies suggesting inverse relation between autophagy and angiogenesis. It is evident by study suggesting that enhanced autophagy blocks angiogenesis in neuroblastoma cells via degradation of gastrin-releasing peptide (GRP). This study suggested use of autophagy activation as novel antivascular therapy in neuroblastomas which are highly vascular in nature (Kim et al. 2013). Another report which shows that silica nanoparticles enhances autophagic activity of endothelial cells and impairs angiogenesis supports the inverse relation between autophagy and angiogenesis (Duan et al. 2014). Activation of AKt/eNOS signalling is reported to inhibit autophagy and enhanced the angiogenesis in cerebral ischemia reperfusion injury (Zheng et al. 2018).

Autophagy's anti-angiogenic effect is also reported to mediate through Wnt/β-Catenin pathway which is a key regulator of angiogenesis, cell proliferation and death (Jiang et al. 2015).

Studies suggest that autophagy has potential to provide both pro-angiogenic and anti-angiogenic response depending on the stimulator or inhibitor of autophagy (Hassanpour, Rezabakhsh, et al. 2018). Autophagy inducers such as triptolid and magnolol depict anti-angiogenic properties (Kumar et al. 2013). They inhibit migration and tube formation of Human Umbilical Vein Endothelial Cells (HUVEC) and apoptotic resistant cancer cells. Although through use of magnolol it was reported that excessive autophagy is responsible for anti-angiogenic effect. This effect could be reversed through blocking of autophagy by 3-MA or *Atg7* and *LC3*gene silencing (Kumar et al. 2013).Excessive autophagy has shown to reduce angiogenic potential in Mesenchymal Stem Cells (MSCs) that are exposed to diabetic serum (Rezabakhsh et al. 2017). These studies suggest relation between autophagy and angiogenesis, but our knowledge lacks in understanding this relation in terms of AD's pathology. There are few studies that indirectly suggest a link between the two in AD. Recent findings reported VEGFR2 decreases in brains of AD mice model and plasma level of VEGFR2 was found to be less in AD patients as compared to healthy controls. Aβ treatment also decreased the gene expression of VEGFR2 in HUVECs (Cho et al. 2017). Another study suggests role of autophagy in direct degradation of VEGFR2 and in impairing angiogenesis in case of diabetes. Expression of VEGFR2 and angiogenesis was reported to decrease in diabetes due to enhanced autophagy (Liu et al. 2012). Although these studies are in different conditions, they suggest that in AD decrease in VEGF due to impaired autophagy and accumulation of Aβ may be responsible for aberrant angiogenesis in AD. Similar to autophagy, mitophagy also has dual effects on angiogenesis. In tumor model mitophagy induction caused decrease in angiogenesis while in other study mitophagy inhibition lead to increase in angiogenesis (Givvimani et al. 2012, Chourasia and Macleod 2015). These studies imply that there is some association between autophagy, mitophagy and angiogenesis in Alzheimer's pathology but it further needs to be explored.

Conclusion

Alzheimer's disease is one of the major neurodegenerative diseases with complex pathology. Beta-amyloid Plaques and abnormal Tau proteins termed as Tau tangles are the pathological hallmarks of AD. Initially it was believed that AD caused degeneration of acetylcholine producing motor neurons only. Later on, it was found that AD can impact other neurotransmitter systems as well. These abnormal proteins exert stress on neurons, microglia and endothelia cells and disrupts proteostatic network over a period of time thereby causing accumulation of protein aggregates. As the autophagy and mitophagy are crucial regulators of proteostasis in cells, their disruption enhances the aggregation of beta plaques and tau tangles. Over a period of time, this biochemical phase of stress leads to cellular phase of AD where inflammatory pathways gets activated leading to chronic inflammation. In the end phase of AD i.e., clinical phase, the cellular homeostasis is completely disrupted causing inexorable disease progression.

Another hallmark of AD is abnormal angiogenesis leading to aberrant vasculature in the brains of AD patients. The enhanced expression of angiogenic factors and their co-localization with Aβ plaques can contribute to the disruption of the normal vasculature. Hypoxia and enhanced ROS also contributes towards the pathophysiology of AD by activating the inflammatory, hypoxic and angiogenic pathways. All of these pathways are also related with autophagy. As discussed in the chapter, there are several reports on the relation between autophagy and angiogenesis is various diseases such as diabetes or cancer. Autophagy can regulate both pro-angiogenic and anti-angiogenic response depending on the stimulator or inhibitor of autophagy. But there is a lack of knowledge regarding the regulation of angiogenesis by autophagy and mitophagy specifically in AD. Exploring the direct relation between autophagy/ mitophagy with angiogenesis and inflammation in AD will pave way for the development of better therapeutic interventions for AD. These interventions will not just be able to control the symptoms of AD but may give rise to complete treatment of AD.

Conflict of Interest

The authors declare that the research was conducted in the absence of any commercial or financial relationships that could be constructed as a potential conflict of interest.

Authors Contribution

S. S. prepared the initial manuscript draft and images. S.J. provided content expertise, overall direction, and reviewed the manuscript. All authors have reviewed the manuscript.

Acknowledgments

We acknowledge the contribution of Indian Institute of Technology Jodhpur and Department of Biotechnology, Government of India for support and funding.

Funding

SJ's laboratory is funded by grants from the Department of Biotechnology (BT/PR12831/MED/30/1489/2015), Government of India and Indian Institute of Technology Jodhpur.

References

Abbott, N Joan, Lars Rönnbäck, and Elisabeth Hansson. 2006. "Astrocyte–endothelial interactions at the blood–brain barrier." *Nature Reviews Neuroscience,* 7 (1):41.

Association, Alzheimer's. 2017. "2017 Alzheimer's disease facts and figures." *Alzheimer's & Dementia*, 13 (4):325-373.

Athanikar, J, LS Perlmutter, D Saperia, and HC Chui. 1988. "Alteration of basement membrane components in dementia." *Society for Neuroscience – Abstracts,* 14:638.

Axe, Elizabeth L, Simon A Walker, Maria Manifava, Priya Chandra, H Llewelyn Roderick, Anja Habermann, Gareth Griffiths, and Nicholas T Ktistakis. 2008. "Autophagosome formation from membrane compartments enriched in phosphatidylinositol 3-phosphate and dynamically connected to the endoplasmic reticulum." *The Journal of Cell Biology,* 182 (4):685-701.

Barker, Warren W, Cheryl A Luis, Alice Kashuba, Mercy Luis, Dylan G Harwood, David Loewenstein, Carol Waters, Pat Jimison, Eugene Shepherd, and Steven Sevush. 2002. "Relative frequencies of Alzheimer disease, Lewy body, vascular and frontotemporal dementia, and hippocampal sclerosis in the State of Florida Brain Bank." *Alzheimer Disease & Associated Disorders,* 16 (4):203-212.

Bastai, P. 1933. "L'involuzione della circolazione capillare considerata come fattore fondamentale della fisiopatologia della vecchiaia." ["The involution of capillary circulation considered as a fundamental factor in the pathophysiology of old age"]. *Minerva Medica,* 24 (2):749-757.

Bateman, Randall J, Chengjie Xiong, Tammie LS Benzinger, Anne M Fagan, Alison Goate, Nick C Fox, Daniel S Marcus, Nigel J Cairns, Xianyun Xie, and Tyler M Blazey. 2012. "Clinical and biomarker changes in dominantly inherited Alzheimer's disease." *New England Journal of Medicine,* 367 (9):795-804.

Bell, Robert D, Rashid Deane, Nienwen Chow, Xiaochun Long, Abhay Sagare, Itender Singh, Jeffrey W Streb, Huang Guo, Anna Rubio, and William Van Nostrand. 2009. "SRF and myocardin regulate LRP-mediated amyloid-β clearance in brain vascular cells." *Nature Cell Biology,* 11 (2):143.

Bellot, Grégory, Raquel Garcia-Medina, Pierre Gounon, Johanna Chiche, Danièle Roux, Jacques Pouysségur, and Nathalie M Mazure. 2009. "Hypoxia-induced autophagy is mediated through hypoxia-inducible factor induction of BNIP3 and BNIP3L via their BH3 domains." *Molecular and Cellular Biology,* 29 (10):2570-2581.

Benarroch, EE. 2007. "Neurovascular unit dysfunction: a vascular component of Alzheimer disease." *Neurology,* 68 (20):1730-1732.

Beskow, J, O Hassler, and J-O Ottosson. 1971. "Cerebral arterial deformities in relation to senile deterioration." *Acta Psychiatrica Scandinavica,* 47 (S221):111-119.

Buee, L, PR Hof, DD Roberts, A Delacourte, JH Morrison, and HM Fillit. 1992. "Immunohistochemical identification of thrombospondin in normal human brain and in Alzheimer's disease." *The American Journal of Pathology,* 141 (4):783.

Calkins, Marcus J, Maria Manczak, Peizhong Mao, Ulziibat Shirendeb, and P Hemachandra Reddy. 2011. "Impaired mitochondrial biogenesis, defective axonal transport of mitochondria, abnormal mitochondrial dynamics and synaptic degeneration in a mouse model of Alzheimer's disease." *Human Molecular Genetics,* 20 (23):4515-4529.

Campbell, A Colin P, Leo Alexander, and Tracy J Putnam. 1938. "Vascular pattern in various lesions of the human central nervous system: Studies with the benzidine stain." *Archives of Neurology & Psychiatry,* 39 (6):1150-1202.

Cataldo, Anne M, Jody L Barnett, Stephen A Berman, Jinhe Li, Shelley Quarless, Sherry Bursztajn, Carol Lippa, and Ralph A Nixon. 1995. "Gene expression and cellular content of cathepsin D in Alzheimer's disease brain: evidence for early up-regulation of the endosomal-lysosomal system." *Neuron,* 14 (3):671-680.

Cataldo, Anne M, Deborah J Hamilton, Jody L Barnett, Peter A Paskevich, and Ralph A Nixon. 1996. "Properties of the endosomal-lysosomal system in the human central nervous system: disturbances mark most neurons in populations at risk to degenerate in Alzheimer's disease." *Journal of Neuroscience,* 16 (1):186-199.

Cerletti, U. 1910. "Die Gefässvermehrung im Zentralnervensystem." ["Vascular proliferation in the central nervous system"]. *Nissl, F., and Alzheimer, A.: Histologie und Histopathologie, Jena, Gustav Fischer,* 4:77.

Chen, Yongshun, Xiaohong Li, Leiming Guo, Xiaoyuan Wu, Chunyu He, Song Zhang, Yanjing Xiao, Yuanyuan Yang, and Daxuan Hao. 2015. "Combining radiation with autophagy inhibition enhances suppression of tumor growth and angiogenesis in esophageal cancer." *Molecular Medicine Reports,* 12 (2):1645-1652.

Cho, Sun-Jung, Moon Ho Park, Changsu Han, Keejung Yoon, and Young Ho Koh. 2017. "VEGFR2 alteration in Alzheimer's disease." *Scientific Reports,* 7 (1):17713.

Chourasia, Aparajita H, and Kay F Macleod. 2015. "Tumor suppressor functions of BNIP3 and mitophagy." *Autophagy,* 11 (10):1937-1938.

Chow, Nienwen, Robert D Bell, Rashid Deane, Jeffrey W Streb, Jiyuan Chen, Andrew Brooks, William Van Nostrand, Joseph M Miano, and Berislav V Zlokovic. 2007. "Serum response factor and myocardin mediate arterial hypercontractility and cerebral blood flow dysregulation in Alzheimer's phenotype." *Proceedings of the National Academy of Sciences,* 104 (3):823-828.

Chu, Charleen T. 2006. "Autophagic stress in neuronal injury and disease." *Journal of Neuropathology & Experimental Neurology,* 65 (5):423-432.

Ciallella, John R, Helmer Figueiredo, Virginia Smith-Swintosky, and Joseph P McGillis. 1999. "Thrombin induces surface and intracellular secretion of amyloid precursor protein from human endothelial cells." *Thrombosis and Haemostasis,* 81 (04):630-637.

Cuervo, Ana Maria. 2010. "Chaperone-mediated autophagy: selectivity pays off." *Trends in Endocrinology & Metabolism,* 21 (3):142-150.

De la Torre, JC, and T Mussivan. 1993. "Can disturbed brain microcirculation cause Alzheimer's disease?" *Neurological Research,* 15 (3):146-153.

De Strooper, Bart, and Eric Karran. 2016. "The cellular phase of Alzheimer's disease." *Cell,* 164 (4):603-615.

Deane, Rashid, Shi Du Yan, Ram Kumar Submamaryan, Barbara LaRue, Suzana Jovanovic, Elizabeth Hogg, Deborah Welch, Lawrence Manness, Chang Lin, and Jin Yu. 2003. "RAGE mediates amyloid-β peptide transport across the blood-brain barrier and accumulation in brain." *Nature Medicine,* 9 (7):907.

Deane, Rashid, Itender Singh, Abhay P Sagare, Robert D Bell, Nathan T Ross, Barbra LaRue, Rachal Love, Sheldon Perry, Nicole Paquette, and Richard J Deane. 2012. "A multimodal RAGE-specific inhibitor reduces amyloid β–mediated brain disorder in a mouse model of Alzheimer disease." *The Journal of Clinical Investigation,* 122 (4):1377-1392.

Deane, Rashid, Zhenhua Wu, and Berislav V Zlokovic. 2004. "RAGE (yin) versus LRP (yang) balance regulates Alzheimer amyloid β-peptide clearance through transport across the blood–brain barrier." *Stroke,* 35 (11_suppl _1):2628-2631.

Deutsch, Georg, and James R Tweedy. 1987. "Cerebral blood flow in severity-matched Alzheimer and multi-infarct patients." *Neurology,* 37 (3):431-431.

Di Meco, Antonio, Mary Elizabeth Curtis, Elisabetta Lauretti, and Domenico Praticó. 2019. "Autophagy dysfunction in Alzheimer's disease: mechanistic insights and new therapeutic opportunities." *Biological Psychiatry,* 87(9) :797-807.

Díaz-Troya, Sandra, María Esther Pérez-Pérez, Francisco J Florencio, and José L Crespo. 2008. "The role of TOR in autophagy regulation from yeast to plants and mammals." *Autophagy,* 4 (7):851-865.

Duan, Junchao, Yongbo Yu, Yang Yu, Yang Li, Peili Huang, Xianqing Zhou, Shuangqing Peng, and Zhiwei Sun. 2014. "Silica nanoparticles enhance autophagic activity, disturb endothelial cell homeostasis and impair angiogenesis." *Particle and Fibre Toxicology,* 11 (1):50.

Fang, Evandro F. 2019. "Mitophagy and NAD+ inhibit Alzheimer disease." *Autophagy,* 15 (6):1112-1114.

Fang, Evandro F, Yujun Hou, Konstantinos Palikaras, Bryan A Adriaanse, Jesse S Kerr, Beimeng Yang, Sofie Lautrup, Md Mahdi Hasan-Olive, Domenica Caponio, and Xiuli Dan. 2019. "Mitophagy inhibits amyloid-β and tau pathology and reverses cognitive deficits in models of Alzheimer's disease." *Nature Neuroscience,* 22 (3):401.

Fetterman, Jessica L, Monica Holbrook, Nir Flint, Bihua Feng, Rosa Bretón-Romero, Erika A Linder, Brittany D Berk, Mai-Ann Duess, Melissa G Farb, and Noyan Gokce. 2016. "Restoration of autophagy in endothelial cells from patients with diabetes mellitus improves nitric oxide signaling." *Atherosclerosis,* 247:207-217.

Filosa, Jessica A, Adrian D Bonev, Stephen V Straub, Andrea L Meredith, M Keith Wilkerson, Richard W Aldrich, and Mark T Nelson. 2006. "Local potassium signaling couples neuronal activity to vasodilation in the brain." *Nature Neuroscience,* 9 (11):1397.

Folin, Marcella, Silvia Baiguera, Diego Guidolin, Rosa Di Liddo, Claudio Grandi, Eugenio De Carlo, Gastone G Nussdorfer, and Pier Paolo Parnigotto. 2006. "Apolipoprotein-E modulates the cytotoxic effect of β-amyloid on rat brain endothelium in an isoform-dependent specific manner." *International Journal of Molecular Medicine,* 17 (5):821-826.

Forette, Françoise, Marie-Laure Seux, Jan A Staessen, Lutgarde Thijs, Willem H Birkenhäger, Marija-Ruta Babarskiene, Speranta Babeanu, Alfredo Bossini, Blas Gil-Extremera, and Xavier Girerd. 1998. "Prevention of dementia in randomised double-blind placebo-controlled Systolic Hypertension in Europe (Syst-Eur) trial." *The Lancet,* 352 (9137):1347-1351.

Friedland, Robert P, Thomas F Budinger, Elisabeth Koss, and Beth A Ober. 1985. "Alzheimer's disease: anterior-posterior and lateral hemispheric alterations in cortical glucose utilization." *Neuroscience Letters,* 53 (3):235-240.

Girouard, Helene, and Costantino Iadecola. 2006. "Neurovascular coupling in the normal brain and in hypertension, stroke, and Alzheimer disease." *Journal of Applied Physiology,* 100 (1):328-335.

Givvimani, Srikanth, Charu Munjal, Neetu Tyagi, Utpal Sen, Naira Metreveli, and Suresh C Tyagi. 2012. "Mitochondrial division/mitophagy inhibitor (Mdivi) ameliorates pressure overload induced heart failure." *PloS One,* 7 (3):e32388.

González-Pecchi, Valentina, Sara Valdés, Véronique Pons, Paula Honorato, Laurent O Martinez, Liliana Lamperti, Claudio Aguayo, and Claudia Radojkovic. 2015. "Apolipoprotein AI enhances proliferation of human endothelial progenitor cells and promotes angiogenesis through the cell surface ATP synthase." *Microvascular Research,* 98:9-15.

Grammas, Paula, and Roma Ovase. 2001. "Inflammatory factors are elevated in brain microvessels in Alzheimer's disease." *Neurobiology of Aging,* 22 (6):837-842.

Hamel, Edith. 2006. "Perivascular nerves and the regulation of cerebrovascular tone." *Journal of Applied Physiology,* 100 (3):1059-1064.

Hassanpour, Mehdi, Omid Cheraghi, Belal Brazvan, Amirataollah Hiradfar, Nasser Aghamohammadzadeh, Reza Rahbarghazi, and Mohammad Nouri. 2018. "Chronic exposure of human endothelial progenitor cells to diabetic condition abolished the regulated kinetics activity of exosomes." *Iranian Journal of Pharmaceutical Research,* 17 (3):1068.

Hassanpour, Mehdi, Aysa Rezabakhsh, Masoud Pezeshkian, Reza Rahbarghazi, and Mohammad Nouri. 2018. "Distinct role of autophagy on angiogenesis: highlights on the effect of autophagy in endothelial lineage and progenitor cells." *Stem Cell Research & Therapy,* 9 (1):305.

Hassler, Ove. 1967. "Arterial deformities in senile brains." *Acta Neuropathologica,* 8 (3):219-229.

Haxby, James V, CL Grady, E Koss, B Horwitz, M Schapiro, RP Friedland, and SI Rapoport. 1988. "Heterogeneous anterior-posterior metabolic patterns in dementia of the Alzheimer type." *Neurology,* 38 (12):1853-1853.

Hayashi, Shin-ichiro, Naoyuki Sato, Akitsugu Yamamoto, Yuka Ikegame, Shigeru Nakashima, Toshio Ogihara, and Ryuichi Morishita. 2009. "Alzheimer disease–associated peptide, amyloid β40, inhibits vascular regeneration with induction of endothelial autophagy." *Arteriosclerosis, Thrombosis, and Vascular Biology,* 29 (11):1909-1915.

He, Congcong, and Daniel J Klionsky. 2009. "Regulation mechanisms and signaling pathways of autophagy." *Annual Review of Genetics,* 43 :67-93.

Higuchi, Yasushi, Taihei Miyakawa, Akitomo Shimoji, and Shoichi Katsuragi. 1987. "Ultrastructural changes of blood vessels in the cerebral cortex in Alzheimer's disease." *Psychiatry and Clinical Neurosciences,* 41 (2):283-290.

Iadecola, Costantino. 2004. "Neurovascular regulation in the normal brain and in Alzheimer's disease." *Nature Reviews Neuroscience,* 5 (5):347.

Iadecola, Costantino, Fangyi Zhang, Kiyoshi Niwa, Chris Eckman, Sherry K Turner, Elizabeth Fischer, Steven Younkin, David R Borchelt, Karen K Hsiao, and George A Carlson. 1999. "SOD1 rescues cerebral endothelial dysfunction in mice overexpressing amyloid precursor protein." *Nature Neuroscience,* 2 (2):157.

In'T Veld, Bas A, Annemieke Ruitenberg, Albert Hofman, Lenore J Launer, Cornelia M van Duijn, Theo Stijnen, Monique MB Breteler, and Bruno HC Stricker. 2001. "Nonsteroidal antiinflammatory drugs and the risk of Alzheimer's disease." *New England Journal of Medicine,* 345 (21):1515-1521.

Inoue, Keiichi, Joanne Rispoli, Hanoch Kaphzan, Eric Klann, Emily I Chen, Jongpil Kim, Masaaki Komatsu, and Asa Abeliovich. 2012. "Macroautophagy deficiency mediates age-dependent neurodegeneration through a phospho-tau pathway." *Molecular Neurodegeneration,* 7 (1):48.

Ivy, GO, F Schottler, J Wenzel, M Baudry, and G Lynch. 1984. "Inhibitors of lysosomal enzymes: accumulation of lipofuscin-like dense bodies in the brain." *Science,* 226 (4677):985-987.

Jiang, Li, Meng Yin, Xiangxiang Wei, Junxu Liu, Xinhong Wang, Cong Niu, Xueling Kang, Jie Xu, Zhongwei Zhou, and Shaoyang Sun. 2015. "Bach1 represses Wnt/β-catenin signaling and angiogenesis." *Circulation Research,* 117 (4):364-375.

Kalaria, RN, DL Cohen, DRD Premkumar, S Nag, JC LaManna, and WD Lust. 1998. "Vascular endothelial growth factor in Alzheimer's disease and experimental cerebral ischemia." *Molecular Brain Research,* 62 (1):101-105.

Karar, Jayashree, and Amit Maity. 2011. "PI3K/AKT/mTOR pathway in angiogenesis." *Frontiers in Molecular Neuroscience,* 4:51.

Katzman, Robert. 1976. "The prevalence and malignancy of Alzheimer disease: a major killer." *Archives of Neurology,* 33 (4):217-218.

Kerr, Jesse S, Bryan A Adriaanse, Nigel H Greig, Mark P Mattson, M Zameel Cader, Vilhelm A Bohr, and Evandro F Fang. 2017. "Mitophagy and Alzheimer's disease: cellular and molecular mechanisms." *Trends in Neurosciences,* 40 (3):151-166.

Kidd, Michael. 1964. "Alzheimer's disease—an electron microscopical study." *Brain,* 87 (2):307-320.

Kim, Kwang Woon, Pritha Paul, Jingbo Qiao, Sora Lee, and Dai H Chung. 2013. "Enhanced autophagy blocks angiogenesis via degradation of gastrin-releasing peptide in neuroblastoma cells." *Autophagy,* 9 (10):1579-1590.

Kimbrough, Ian F, Stefanie Robel, Erik D Roberson, and Harald Sontheimer. 2015. "Vascular amyloidosis impairs the gliovascular unit in a mouse model of Alzheimer's disease." *Brain,* 138 (12):3716-3733.

Kisler, Kassandra, Amy R Nelson, Axel Montagne, and Berislav V Zlokovic. 2017. "Cerebral blood flow regulation and neurovascular dysfunction in Alzheimer disease." *Nature Reviews Neuroscience,* 18 (7):419.

Klionsky, Daniel J, Eric H Baehrecke, John H Brumell, Charleen T Chu, Patrice Codogno, Ana Maria Cuervo, Jayanta Debnath, Vojo Deretic, Zvulun Elazar, and Eeva-Liisa Eskelinen. 2011. "A comprehensive glossary of autophagy-related molecules and processes." *Autophagy,* 7 (11):1273-1294.

Koehler, Raymond C, Debebe Gebremedhin, and David R Harder. 2006. "Role of astrocytes in cerebrovascular regulation." *Journal of Applied Physiology,* 100 (1):307-317.

Koike, Masato, Hiroshi Nakanishi, Paul Saftig, Junji Ezaki, Kyoko Isahara, Yoshiyuki Ohsawa, Walter Schulz-Schaeffer, Tsuyoshi Watanabe, Satoshi Waguri, and Satoshi Kametaka. 2000. "Cathepsin D deficiency induces lysosomal storage with ceroid lipofuscin in mouse CNS neurons." *Journal of Neuroscience,* 20 (18):6898-6906.

Kumar, S, SK Guru, AS Pathania, A Kumar, S Bhushan, and F Malik. 2013. "Autophagy triggered by magnolol derivative negatively regulates angiogenesis." *Cell Death & Disease,* 4 (10):e889.

Kurtishi, Alberim, Benjamin Rosen, Ketan S Patil, Guido W Alves, and Simon G Møller. 2019. "Cellular proteostasis in neurodegeneration." *Molecular Neurobiology,* 56 (5):3676-3689.

Labbadia, Johnathan, and Richard I Morimoto. 2015. "The biology of proteostasis in aging and disease." *Annual Review of Biochemistry,* 84:435-464.

Lee, Ju-Hyun, W Haung Yu, Asok Kumar, Sooyeon Lee, Panaiyur S Mohan, Corrinne M Peterhoff, Devin M Wolfe, Marta Martinez-Vicente, Ashish C Massey, and Guy Sovak. 2010. "Lysosomal proteolysis and autophagy require presenilin 1 and are disrupted by Alzheimer-related PS1 mutations." *Cell,* 141 (7):1146-1158.

Lesniewski, Lisa A, Douglas R Seals, Ashley E Walker, Grant D Henson, Mark W Blimline, Daniel W Trott, Gary C Bosshardt, Thomas J LaRocca, Brooke R Lawson, and Melanie C Zigler. 2017. "Dietary rapamycin supplementation reverses age-related vascular dysfunction and oxidative stress, while modulating nutrient-sensing, cell cycle, and senescence pathways." *Aging Cell,* 16 (1):17-26.

Lin, Ai-Ling, Wei Zheng, Jonathan J Halloran, Raquel R Burbank, Stacy A Hussong, Matthew J Hart, Martin Javors, Yen-Yu Ian Shih, Eric Muir, and Rene Solano Fonseca. 2013. "Chronic rapamycin restores brain vascular integrity and function through NO synthase activation and improves memory in symptomatic mice modeling Alzheimer's disease." *Journal of Cerebral Blood Flow & Metabolism,* 33 (9):1412-1421.

Liu, Hongtao, Shujie Yu, Hua Zhang, and Jian Xu. 2012. "Angiogenesis impairment in diabetes: role of methylglyoxal-induced receptor for advanced glycation endproducts, autophagy and vascular endothelial growth factor receptor 2." *PloS One,* 7 (10):e46720.

Liu, Hui, Hongyan Qiu, Qian Xiao, and Weidong Le. 2015. "Chronic hypoxia-induced autophagy aggravates the neuropathology of Alzheimer's disease through AMPK-mTOR signaling in the APP swe/PS1 dE9 mouse model." *Journal of Alzheimer's Disease,* 48 (4):1019-1032.

Mancardi, GL, F Perdelli, C Rivano, A Leonardi, and O Bugiani. 1980. "Thickening of the basement membrane of cortical capillaries in Alzheimer's disease." *Acta Neuropathologica,* 49 (1):79-83.

Manczak, Maria, Marcus J Calkins, and P Hemachandra Reddy. 2011. "Impaired mitochondrial dynamics and abnormal interaction of amyloid beta with mitochondrial protein Drp1 in neurons from patients with Alzheimer's disease: implications for neuronal damage." *Human Molecular Genetics,* 20 (13):2495-2509.

Manczak, Maria, and P Hemachandra Reddy. 2012. "Abnormal interaction between the mitochondrial fission protein Drp1 and hyperphosphorylated tau in Alzheimer's disease neurons: implications for mitochondrial dysfunction and neuronal damage." *Human Molecular Genetics,* 21 (11):2538-2547.

Marco, Sonia, and Stephen D Skaper. 2006. "Amyloid β-peptide1–42 alters tight junction protein distribution and expression in brain microvessel endothelial cells." *Neuroscience Letters,* 401 (3):219-224.

Mathys, Hansruedi, Jose Davila-Velderrain, Zhuyu Peng, Fan Gao, Shahin Mohammadi, Jennie Z Young, Madhvi Menon, Liang He, Fatema Abdurrob, and Xueqiao Jiang. 2019. "Single-cell transcriptomic analysis of Alzheimer's disease." *Nature*, 570 :332-337.

McGeer, Patrick L, Michael Schulzer, and Edith G McGeer. 1996. "Arthritis and anti-inflammatory agents as possible protective factors for Alzheimer's disease: a review of 17 epidemiologic studies." *Neurology,* 47 (2):425-432.

Miyakawa, T, S Katsuragi, K Watanabe, A Shimoji, and Y Ikeuchi. 1986. "Ultrastructural studies of amyloid fibrils and senile plaques in human brain." *Acta Neuropathologica,* 70 (3-4):202-208.

Miyakawa, Taihei, and Ryoko Kuramoto. 1989. "Ultrastructural study of senile plaques and microvessels in the brain with Alzheimer's disease and Down's syndrome." *Annals of Medicine,* 21 (2):99-102.

Miyakawa, Taihei, and Yasuo Uehara. 1979. "Observations of amyloid angiopathy and senile plaques by the scanning electron microscope." *Acta Neuropathologica,* 48 (2):153-156.

Mizushima, Noboru, Beth Levine, Ana Maria Cuervo, and Daniel J Klionsky. 2008. "Autophagy fights disease through cellular self-digestion." *Nature,* 451 (7182):1069.

Nilsson, Per, Krishnapriya Loganathan, Misaki Sekiguchi, Yukio Matsuba, Kelvin Hui, Satoshi Tsubuki, Motomasa Tanaka, Nobuhisa Iwata, Takashi Saito, and Takaomi C Saido. 2013. "Aβ secretion and plaque formation depend on autophagy." *Cell Reports,* 5 (1):61-69.

Nixon, Ralph A. 2013. "The role of autophagy in neurodegenerative disease." *Nature Medicine,* 19 (8):983.

Nixon, Ralph A, and Anne M Cataldo. 2006. "Lysosomal system pathways: genes to neurodegeneration in Alzheimer's disease." *Journal of Alzheimer's Disease,* 9 (s3):277-289.

Nixon, Ralph A, Jerzy Wegiel, Asok Kumar, Wai Haung Yu, Corrinne Peterhoff, Anne Cataldo, and Ana Maria Cuervo. 2005. "Extensive involvement of autophagy in Alzheimer disease: an immuno-electron microscopy study." *Journal of Neuropathology & Experimental Neurology,* 64 (2):113-122.

Nixon, Ralph A, and Dun-Sheng Yang. 2011. "Autophagy failure in Alzheimer's disease—locating the primary defect." *Neurobiology of Disease,* 43 (1):38-45.

Ntsapi, Claudia, Dumisile Lumkwana, Chrisna Swart, Andre du Toit, and Ben Loos. 2018. "New insights into autophagy dysfunction related to amyloid beta toxicity and neuropathology in Alzheimer's disease." *International Review of Cell and Molecular Biology*, 336 » 321-361.

Oliver, Darryll MA, and P Hemachandra Reddy. 2019. "Small molecules as therapeutic drugs for Alzheimer's disease." *Molecular and Cellular Neuroscience*, 96 :47-62.

Palop, Jorge J, and Lennart Mucke. 2010. "Amyloid-β–induced neuronal dysfunction in Alzheimer's disease: from synapses toward neural networks." *Nature Neuroscience,* 13 (7):812.

Papassotiropoulos, Andreas, Metin Bagli, Alexander Kurz, Johannes Kornhuber, Hans Förstl, Wolfgang Maier, Jutta Pauls, Nicola Lautenschlager, and Reinhard Heun. 2000. "A genetic variation of cathepsin D is a major risk factor for Alzheimer's disease." *Annals of Neurology: Official Journal of the American Neurological Association and the Child Neurology Society,* 47 (3):399-403.

Park, Laibaik, Josef Anrather, Ping Zhou, Kelly Frys, Rose Pitstick, Steven Younkin, George A Carlson, and Costantino Iadecola. 2005. "NADPH oxidase-derived reactive oxygen species mediate the cerebrovascular dysfunction induced by the amyloid β peptide." *Journal of Neuroscience,* 25 (7):1769-1777.

Park, Laibaik, Kenzo Koizumi, Sleiman El Jamal, Ping Zhou, Mary Lou Previti, William E Van Nostrand, George Carlson, and Costantino Iadecola. 2014. "Age-dependent neurovascular dysfunction and damage in a mouse model of cerebral amyloid angiopathy." *Stroke,* 45 (6):1815-1821.

Park, Laibaik, Gang Wang, Ping Zhou, Joan Zhou, Rose Pitstick, Mary Lou Previti, Linda Younkin, Steven G Younkin, William E Van Nostrand, and Sunghee Cho. 2011. "Scavenger receptor CD36 is essential for the cerebrovascular oxidative stress and neurovascular dysfunction induced by amyloid-β." *Proceedings of the National Academy of Sciences,* 108 (12):5063-5068.

Park, SY, MY Park, HG Park, KJ Lee, MS Kook, WJ Kim, and JY Jung. 2017. "Nitric oxide-induced autophagy and the activation of activated protein kinase pathway protect against apoptosis in human dental pulp cells." *International Endodontic Journal,* 50 (3):260-270.

Perlmutter, LS, J Athanikar, C Zarow, and HC Chui. 1988. "Basement membrane pathology in dementia." *Society for Neuroscience - Abstracts.*

Perlmutter, Lynn S, Helena C Chui, David Saperia, and Jyoti Athanikar. 1990. "Microangiopathy and the colocalization of heparan sulfate proteoglycan with amyloid in senile plaques of Alzheimer's disease." *Brain Research,* 508 (1):13-19.

Piras, Antonio, Ludovic Collin, Fiona Grüninger, Caroline Graff, and Annica Rönnbäck. 2016. "Autophagic and lysosomal defects in human tauopathies: analysis of post-mortem brain from patients with familial Alzheimer disease, corticobasal degeneration and progressive supranuclear palsy." *Acta Neuropathologica Communications,* 4 (1):22.

Ravens, JR. 1978. "Vascular changes in the human senile brain." *Advances in Neurology* 20:487.

Reddy, P Hemachandra. 2006. "Mitochondrial oxidative damage in aging and Alzheimer's disease: implications for mitochondrially targeted antioxidant therapeutics." *BioMed Research International.*

Reddy, P Hemachandra, Shannon McWeeney, Byung S Park, Maria Manczak, Ramana V Gutala, Dara Partovi, Youngsin Jung, Vincent Yau, Robert Searles, and Motomi Mori. 2004. "Gene expression profiles of transcripts in amyloid precursor protein transgenic mice: up-regulation of mitochondrial metabolism and apoptotic genes is an early cellular change in Alzheimer's disease." *Human Molecular Genetics,* 13 (12):1225-1240.

Reddy, P Hemachandra, and Darryll Oliver. 2019. "Amyloid beta and phosphorylated tau-induced defective autophagy and mitophagy in alzheimer's disease." *Cells,* 8 (5):488.

Rezabakhsh, Aysa, Omid Cheraghi, Alireza Nourazarian, Mehdi Hassanpour, Masoumeh Kazemi, Shahrooz Ghaderi, Esmaeil Faraji, Reza Rahbarghazi, Çığır Biray Avci, and Bakiye Goker Bagca. 2017. "Type 2 diabetes inhibited human mesenchymal stem cells angiogenic response by over-activity of the autophagic pathway." *Journal of Cellular Biochemistry,* 118 (6):1518-1530.

Rossi, David J. 2006. "Another BOLD role for astrocytes: coupling blood flow to neural activity." *Nature Neuroscience,* 9 (2):159.

Sagare, Abhay P, Robert D Bell, Zhen Zhao, Qingyi Ma, Ethan A Winkler, Anita Ramanathan, and Berislav V Zlokovic. 2013. "Pericyte loss influences Alzheimer-like neurodegeneration in mice." *Nature Communications,* 4:2932.

Scheibel, Arnold B, Taihung Duong, and Roland Jacobs. 1989. "Alzheimer's disease as a capillary dementia." *Annals of Medicine,* 21 (2):103-107.

Scheibel, Arnold B, Adam F Wechsler, and Mary Agnes Burniston Brazier. 1986. "The biological substrates of Alzheimer's disease." Orlando : Academic Press.

Selkoe, Dennis J. 2001. "Alzheimer's disease: genes, proteins, and therapy." *Physiological Review,s* 81 (2):741-766.

Siedlak, Sandra L, Patrick Cras, Mitsuru Kawai, Peggy Richey, and George Perry. 1991. "Basic fibroblast growth factor binding is a marker for extracellular neurofibrillary tangles in Alzheimer disease." *Journal of Histochemistry & Cytochemistry,* 39 (7):899-904.

Suzuki, Yoshio, Shin-Ichi Satoh, Ichiro Ikegaki, Tomohisa Okada, Masato Shibuya, Kenichiro Sugita, and Toshio Asano. 1989. "Effects of neuropeptide Y and calcitonin gene-related peptide on local cerebral blood flow in rat striatum." *Journal of Cerebral Blood Flow & Metabolism,* 9 (3):268-270.

Tagliavini, F, J Ghiso, WF Timmers, G Giaccone, O Bugiani, and B Frangione. 1990. "Coexistence of Alzheimer's amyloid precursor protein and amyloid protein in cerebral vessel walls." *Laboratory Investigation; A Journal of Technical Methods and Pathology,* 62 (6):761-767.

Tammineni, Prasad, Xuan Ye, Tuancheng Feng, Daniyal Aikal, and Qian Cai. 2017. "Impaired retrograde transport of axonal autophagosomes contributes to autophagic stress in Alzheimer's disease neurons." *eLife,* 6:e21776.

Tarkowski, Elisabeth, Razao Issa, Magnus Sjögren, Anders Wallin, Kaj Blennow, Andrej Tarkowski, and Pat Kumar. 2002. "Increased intrathecal levels of the angiogenic factors VEGF and TGF-β in Alzheimer's disease and vascular dementia." *Neurobiology of Aging,* 23 (2):237-243.

Torisu, Takehiro, Kumiko Torisu, In Hye Lee, Jie Liu, Daniela Malide, Christian A Combs, Xufeng S Wu, Ilsa I Rovira, Maria M Fergusson, and Roberto Weigert. 2013. "Autophagy regulates endothelial cell processing, maturation and secretion of von Willebrand factor." *Nature Medicine,* 19 (10):1281.

Tuke, J Batty. 1873. "On the morbid histology of the brain and spinal cord as observed in the insane." *The British and Foreign Medico-Chirurgical Review,* 51 (102):450.

Uddin, Md Sahab, Abdullah Al Mamun, Zubair Khalid Labu, Oscar Hidalgo-Lanussa, George E Barreto, and Ghulam Md Ashraf. 2019. "Autophagic dysfunction in Alzheimer's disease: cellular and molecular mechanistic approaches to halt Alzheimer's pathogenesis." *Journal of Cellular Physiology,* 234 (6):8094-8112.

Uddin, Md, Anna Stachowiak, Abdullah Al Mamun, Nikolay T Tzvetkov, Shinya Takeda, Atanas G Atanasov, Leandro B Bergantin, Mohamed M Abdel-Daim, and Adrian M Stankiewicz. 2018. "Autophagy and Alzheimer's disease: from molecular mechanisms to therapeutic implications." *Frontiers in Aging Neuroscience,* 10:4.

Vagnucci Jr, Anthony H, and William W Li. 2003. "Alzheimer's disease and angiogenesis." *The Lancet,* 361 (9357):605-608.

Valentijn, Karine M, J Evan Sadler, Jack A Valentijn, Jan Voorberg, and Jeroen Eikenboom. 2011. "Functional architecture of Weibel-Palade bodies." *Blood,* 117 (19):5033-5043.

Villemagne, Victor L, Samantha Burnham, Pierrick Bourgeat, Belinda Brown, Kathryn A Ellis, Olivier Salvado, Cassandra Szoeke, S Lance Macaulay, Ralph Martins, and Paul Maruff. 2013. "Amyloid β deposition, neurodegeneration, and cognitive decline in sporadic Alzheimer's disease: a prospective cohort study." *The Lancet Neurology,* 12 (4):357-367.

Vissers, Caroline, Guo-li Ming, and Hongjun Song. 2019. "Nanoparticle technology and stem cell therapy team up against neurodegenerative disorders." *Advanced Drug Delivery Reviews*, 148 :239-251.

Wilhelmus, Micha MM, Irene Otte-Höller, Jos JJ Van Triel, Robert Veerhuis, Marion LC Maat-Schieman, Guojun Bu, Robert MW De Waal, and Marcel M Verbeek. 2007. "Lipoprotein receptor-related protein-1 mediates amyloid-β-mediated cell death of cerebrovascular cells." *The American Journal of Pathology,* 171 (6):1989-1999.

Wilson, Robert S, Eisuke Segawa, Patricia A Boyle, Sophia E Anagnos, Loren P Hizel, and David A Bennett. 2012. "The natural history of cognitive decline in Alzheimer's disease." *Psychology and Aging,* 27 (4):1008.

Wolfe, Devin M, Ju-hyun Lee, Asok Kumar, Sooyeon Lee, Samantha J Orenstein, and Ralph A Nixon. 2013. "Autophagy failure in A lzheimer's disease and the role of defective lysosomal acidification." *European Journal of Neuroscience,* 37 (12):1949-1961.

Wong, Esther, and Ana Maria Cuervo. 2010. "Autophagy gone awry in neurodegenerative diseases." *Nature Neuroscience,* 13 (7):805.

Wu, Min Huan, Chih-Yang Huang, JA Lin, Shih-Wei Wang, Chieh-Yu Peng, Hsu-Chen Cheng, and Chih-Hsin Tang. 2014. "Endothelin-1 promotes vascular endothelial growth factor-dependent angiogenesis in human chondrosarcoma cells." *Oncogene,* 33 (13):1725.

Xie, Zhiping, and Daniel J Klionsky. 2007. "Autophagosome formation: core machinery and adaptations." *Nature Cell Biology,* 9 (10):1102.

Yang, Seung-Pil, Dong-Goo Bae, Hyo Jung Kang, Byoung Joo Gwag, Yong Song Gho, and Chi-Bom Chae. 2004. "Co-accumulation of vascular endothelial growth factor with β-amyloid in the brain of patients with Alzheimer's disease." *Neurobiology of Aging,* 25 (3):283-290.

Zheng, Yongqiu, Zhenzhen Wu, Frank Yi, Matthew Orange, Mingjiang Yao, Bin Yang, Jianxun Liu, and Hua Zhu. 2018. "By activating Akt/eNOS Bilobalide B inhibits autophagy and promotes angiogenesis following focal cerebral ischemia reperfusion." *Cellular Physiology and Biochemistry,* 47 (2):604-616.

Ziche, Marina, Lucia Morbidelli, Emanuela Masini, Sandra Amerini, Harris J Granger, Carlo Alberto Maggi, Pierangelo Geppetti, and Fabrizio Ledda. 1994. "Nitric oxide mediates angiogenesis in vivo and endothelial cell growth and migration in vitro promoted by substance P." *The Journal of Clinical Investigation,* 94 (5):2036-2044.

Zlokovic, Berislav V. 2005. "Neurovascular mechanisms of Alzheimer's neuro-degeneration." *Trends in Neurosciences,* 28 (4):202-208.

Chapter 9

Neuro-Nanotechnology: A Boon to Neurosurgery

Apoorva Kumar*
Department of Advanced Neurosurgery, Charak Hospital,
Lucknow, Uttar Pradesh, India

Abstract

Nanotechnology is among the fast and rapidly growing fields of science, engineering and technology and it has also revolutionized the health sector. Among these it has countless amazing features in area of neurosurgery. In recent years, surgeons in the area of neuroscience are successfully using various nanotechnology-based devices, materials, drugs and techniques in their surgery as per requirements. Therefore, this chapter highlights the several usages and applications of nanotechnology in neuro-surgery with remarkable research studies.

Introduction

Nanotechnology is an emerging field of science and engineering that uses new tools and approaches in concern to apply, design, synthesize and characterize the material and devices that are capable of interacting with cell and tissues at molecular and subcellular level having functional organization of at least 1 dimension on the nanometre. It includes countless features of technology including neurosurgery [1]. Nanotechnology is a high interdisciplinary area of

---

* Corresponding Author's Email: Apoorvakumar80@gmail.com.

In: New Perspectives in Neuroscience
Editors: Prachi Srivastava, Neha Srivastava and Prekshi Garg
ISBN: 978-1-68507-754-9

research and development in concurrence with basic and clinical neuroscience including molecular biology, neurophysiology as well as neuropathology along with integration of chemistry and material science with specific nano-approaches to the nervous system. In recent years, neurosurgeons are actively utilizing nanotechnologies [2] in providing better research strategies for utmost clinical applicability of nano-engineered devices, material or drugs at the brain of patients according to needs. The advancement of technology in neurosurgery should be focused on two strategies: nano-manipulation, nano-imaging and nano-neuromodulation.

Nano-manipulation techniques refers to the surgery performed on the brain at the degree of neuronal and intracellular processes in order to restore the functional regeneration as well as protection of the nervous system after degenerative insult or traumatic brain injury.

Nano-imaging refers to the ability of visualizing the nervous system and cellular and subcellular level. The non-surgical nano-repair techniques not only advance the axonal regeneration and haemorrhage blocking, but also provide therapeutic solutions to the various neurological deficits after post brain tumour treatment, trauma and stroke.

Nano-neuromodulation refers to pain management in patients suffering from neuropathic or cancer. Moreover, it also helps in blocking NMDA receptors or local sensorial circuits by releasing catecholamine and opioid peptides [3].

Nanotools for Neuroscience and Neurosurgery

The biggest challenge of nanoscience is to understand the insight of the neuron process and integrate synaptic input and also the mechanism of brain activities. With the rapid advancement in field neuro-nanotechnology, has shown-up new possibilities to tackle these challenges and develop novel therapeutic intervention for neurological deficits. Therefore, in this chapter we will in detail summarize the various roles and significance of neuro-nanotechnology in understanding the central nervous system (CNS) function and disorders. In addition, we will also discuss the applicability of nanotools in neurosurgery.

Imaging Nanotools

In the 1940s and 60s, nanotechnology was merely based on microscopic techniques including scanning tunnelling microscope (STM), the transmission electron microscope (TEM), and the scanning electron microscope (SEM) that was used to resolve images on nano-scale at high resolution. Later on, atomic force microscopy (AFM) was invented that was able to resolve nano topography of surfaces and project the physico-chemical forces of the spatial distributions [4]. Moreover, in the past decade, the microscopic techniques rapidly improved with advancement in confocal microscopy and total internal reflection fluorescence microscopy (TIRFM) techniques. In recent years, the nano-scale tools have shown their greatest potential in visualizing not only cellular structures but also macro-molecular structures as well. In addition, they are also used in rapid evaluation of nano-scale dynamics at a single molecular level. The introduction of the Stimulated Emission Depletion (STED) microscopy brings revolution in microscopy techniques, and is used to achieve resolution below the diffraction limits. STED generates a maximum resolution of 20-50 nm. It is used to image cellular microcosmos of the nanoscale topology. The optical imaging tools PALM [6] and STORM [7] having nanoscale resolution aid scientists to study nanoscale objects within the cell with maximum resolution of ~20 nm or better spatial precision. These techniques showed their potential in unveiling the macromolecular complexes architect within the specialized cell of the nervous system [8]. A study based on these techniques reveals the dynamic organization of actin cytoskeleton with the cell which suggest the role of neuron probe in neuronal growth and injury and also how it evolves axonal process [9]. Furthermore, these techniques also help in understanding the stereochemistry and clustering of receptors in plasma membranes under certain conditions [10, 11] as well as in understanding the organisation of protein inside the synapse which is crucial for examining the response of synapses while the neuronal changes [12].

Nanoparticles

Nanoparticles, a notable nanotechnology-based tool that is regularly used in neuroscience research and neurosurgery as well. One of the magnificent features are the Quantum Dots [13]. These semiconductor nanoparticles have distinctive electronic and optical features such as photobleaching resistance, high quantum yields, narrow spectrum emission, used for high resolution imaging and labelling of probes in specific molecules and biological tissues [14]. Alongside the DNA Nanotechnology used in synthesis of artificial nucleic acid and nanomaterials including fullerenes [15], CNTs [16], graphene [17] for technological applications. Amid several promising nano tools, colloidal gold Nanoparticles (AuNPs) have salient features such as diameter of wide range from 5-400 nm, interaction with visible light with varieties of emission spectra useful in microscopy and bioimaging. It has been also used as drug-delivery agent and as sensor in diagnostic application. The study suggested the ability of AuNPs to convert light into heat indicating it's the characteristics as neuronal stimulation technique [18]. This novel technique allows light-driven neuronal stimulation without viral transduction with minimal invasion in comparison to electrophysiology. Another promising tool in neurosurgery is magnetic particle imaging (MPI). The MPI is a radiation free tomographic method that provides direct spatial distribution on SPIONS in a biological specimen with high spatial and temporal resolution along with utmost sensitivity shows promising role in detecting various neurosurgical diseases including primary brain tumour associated with hematoma, traumatic brain injury [19].

Neuro Drug Delivery System

Due to the versatile feature of nanoparticles, it can be employed in numerous applications of medical and health sciences. With the advent of nanotechnology lead towards the efficient way of drug delivery to the brain and across the blood brain barrier (BBB) as well. In brain parenchyma the poorly distributed drugs have higher druggable bioactivity which on upload to the nanocarrier system shows good interaction with endothelial micro-vessel cells. These nanocarriers are active with target ligands showing picky binding with a receptor or transporter expressed in BBB which increase the permeability and selectivity of CNS [20]. Solid lipid nanoparticles (SLNP) are used as a drug carrier to deliver drugs to the brain in cancer patients [21]. Quercetin, a novel neuroprotectant, inhibits the overproduction of reactive oxygen species generated by mitochondrial dysfunction in Alzheimer patients. The study reported [22] the use of microencapsulation techniques by the formulation of SLNP with surfactant Tween 80 and lipid camphritol enhance the delivery of Quercetin in brain. Further the finding suggested the improved memory retention in rats with quercetin in comparison to without quercetin. Moreover, the target specific drug delivery system is also being designed as a therapeutic strategy such as in Glioblastoma multiforme (GBM), a grade 4 malignant brain cancer. The study suggested the inhibition of grade 4 glioma by encapsulating the carmustine in catatonic SLNP with anti-epithelial growth factor receptors. In continuation, the nanoparticles efficiently deliver the drug into U87MG cells and enhance the anticancer activity against the brain tumor based on concentration of surfactant [23].

Nanodevices in Neurological Surgery Procedures

Nanoscale based new micro-fabricated devices featuring as a new micro instrument for neuro-surgical procedures. The carbon nanostructure-like neuritis having outstanding electrical, mechanical and conduction properties [24], due to which they have been employed to enhance the neural activities and to guide severed ends of nerves [25]. There could also be chances of various surface changes on MWCNTs via chemical functionalization which in turn are a controlling factor for nerve growth. The activation of phospholipase-C pathway has also been reported in nerve growth factor treated neurons by carbon nanotubes [26].

The recent advancement in the field of nanotechnology has resulted in the development of non-invasive minimal access surgery. The nano-robotics technology has made it possible that now a nano-robot can be injected into a patient to perform a particular diagnosis or treatment which takes place at a cellular nano-scale level [27]. Magnetic nanobots are used to safely deliver drug molecules across the blood-brain barrier via hyperthermic disruption of the blood-brain barrier by inducting MNPs inside an AC field [28]. The efficiency of these robots depends on the precision with which the motion controllers are conjugated in it [29]. Employing this hypothesis, a magnetotactic bacterium (MTB) is controlled by controlling the orientation of the magnetic field and positioning it towards the target in an attempt to enhance the drug delivery [30]. Two photon polymerizations were utilized to manufacture a controllable activated swimming nano-robots made of a magnetic polymer composite (MPC) containing magnetite nanoparticles of 11 nm in distance across and photograph treatable resin [31]. Similarly, neuro-intrusive multi-designated drug conveyance was accomplished utilizing a multitude of attractive nanorobots carriers [32]. Similar reports on drug conveyance utilizing nanorobots were depicted somewhere else.

Concerning the trouble experienced by neurosurgeons during growth medical procedure, the utilization of nano surgery is hailed as a magnificent use of nanotechnology to the field of neuromedicine. During this sort of surgery, the growths are controlled or quenched by coordinating light emissions quick laser radiates that are engaged by a genuine magnifying lens focal point. Ben-Yakar and Bourgeois [33] announced the utilization of ultrafast laser nano surgery for *in vivo* nerve recovery studies. Femtosecond laser beats was displayed to give the original ability to exact, sub-surface, cell scale cuts for neurosurgical applications in rats [34]. Also, a clever photo disruption strategy portrayed as Plasmonic Laser Nano-surgery (PLN) was utilized to takes advantage of the huge upgrade of ultrafast laser beats in the close field of gold nanoparticles for the nanoscale control of natural structures [35]. Recent systems concerning clinical laser medical procedure were assessed in some literatures [36, 37].

For more than fifty years, changed protected microelectrodes were known to be utilized in neurophysiological studies [38]. Previously it has been revealed the utilization of silicon substrate microelectrode arrays embedded in cerebral cortex for constant cerebrum cortical recording [39]. Qiao et al. [40] exhibited that 700 nm tipped anode recorded very much disengaged activity possibilities extracellularly from single visual neurons in vivo. Further trial concentrates on utilizing sub-100 nm silicon nanowires uncovered its combination into live cells without causing impeding effects [41]. Transistor varieties of silicon nanowires with breadth of 30 nm that were created on straightforward substrates were utilized to plan neural circuits in intense cerebrum cuts (Qing et al. 2010). The neural circuit is said to give a road that can record across a wide scope of length scales, while the straightforward gadget chips just give imaging of individual cell bodies [38]. Recently, Robinson et al. [42] portrayed a versatile stage for intracellular interfacing to neuronal circuits utilizing vertical nanowire cathode clusters. The mix of exhibits with fixed clasp was utilized to record the action with a high worldly and spatial goal, just as planning of useful availability, giving an amazing stage to concentrating on neural circuits in the mind.

Accuracy is viewed as one of the utmost significant elements in surgeries including neurosurgery, and the mechanical technology commitment of nanotechnology has presented one more aspect in the field of neurosurgery. Nanorobots scaled down nanoscale gadgets manufactured from dynamic nanomaterials, for example, engineered zinc oxide, gold, quartz and so forth are said to fill in as sensors and additionally actuators that can be utilized in negligible access or nanoscale surgeries with unrivalled precision [43-45]. The PC directed calculations of this sort of advanced mechanics assist the specialist with definitively directing the robot to an area at a sub-nanometre or nanometre goal, making it conceivable to see neurological illness areas that could be difficult to see before [46]. Recently, a clever picture directed framework has been created for exact, programmed focusing of designs inside the brain [47]. The creators detailed the robots to either be added straightforwardly to a head clasp or to the patient skull along the course of a medical procedure. Once positioned, it naturally positions itself with incredible accuracy. Utilizing modified data acquired from preoperative electronic sweeps of the patient, the small robots are fit for focusing on mind growths with an accuracy that has never been. Likewise, SpineAssist® a small bone-mounted mechanical framework for insignificantly obtrusive spinal medical procedure was created in the equivalent laboratory [48]. The robot is said to have a general accuracy of around 1 mm during pedicle screw in both open and negligibly intrusive strategies. Another clever nanotechnology that will clearly reform the period of negligible access neurosurgical methodology is the "telerobotic medical procedure" utilizing Robot-Assisted Microsurgery (RAMS) [49]. The trustworthiness and accuracy of this innovation was analysed by Le Roux et al. [50] against the customary microsurgical methods in making and shutting carotid arteriotomies in rodents. The creators noticed the strategies to be like customary microsurgical methods as far as execution mistake, accuracy, and specialized quality [51].

Conclusion

Nanotechnology, as we all know by now, is an emerging field and also versatile in application. It has emerged as an amazing aid in surgery and medical treatment procedures, from diagnosis to cure. The association of nanotechnology and surgery is surely a boon in many ways, from enhanced drug delivery systems to targeted therapies and also this association allows surgeons to non-invasively access the deepest tissue and tumours. Concerning the trouble experienced by neurosurgeons during growth medical procedure, the utilization of nano surgery is hailed as a magnificent use of nanotechnology to the field of neuromedicine. The use of CNTs, MWCNTs, nano-bots, magnetic nanorobots and many other specialized devices in neurosurgery is advancing day by day and this is a step ahead in the direction of personalized medicine.

References

[1] Russell JA. (2009). Nanotechnology and neurosurgery. *Journal of Neuroscience and Nanotechnology*, 9:5008-5013.

[2] Saini R, Saini S. (2010). Nanotechnology and surgical neurology. *Surgical Neurology International*, 1:57-57.

[3] Iacob G, Ciurea AV. Ed. Universitara Carol Davila; București (2003). Curs de tehnici neurochirurgicale în tratamentul durerii cornice [*Carol Davila University; Bucharest (2003). Course in neurosurgical techniques in the treatment of chronic pain*]; pp. 195-196.

[4] Pampaloni Niccolò Paolo, Giugliano Michele, Scaini Denis, Ballerini Laura, Rauti Rossana. (2019) Advances in Nano Neuroscience: From Nanomaterials to Nanotools. *Frontiers in Neuroscience*, 12,953,SSN= 1662-453X.

[5] Hell, S. W., and Wichmann, J. (1994). Breaking the diffraction resolution limit by stimulated emission: stimulated-emission-depletion fluorescence microscopy. *Optics Letters*, 19, 780-782. doi: 10.1364/OL.19.000780.

[6] Pisanello, F., Sileo, L., and De Vittorio, M. (2016). Micro- and nanotechnologies for optical neural interfaces. *Frontiers in Neurosci*ence. 10:70. doi: 10.3389/fnins.2 016.00070.

[7] Rust, M. J., Bates, M., and Zhuang, X. W. (2006). Sub-diffraction-limit imaging by stochastic optical reconstruction microscopy (STORM). *Nature Methods,* 3, 793-795. doi: 10.1038/nmeth929.

[8] Alivisatos, A. P., Andrews, A. M., Boyden, E. S., Chun, M., Church, G. M., Deisseroth, K., et al. (2013). Nanotools for neuroscience and brain activity mapping. *ACS Nano*, 7, 1850-1866. doi: 10.1021/nn4012847.

[9] Xu, K., Zhong, G., and Zhuang, X. (2013). Actin, spectrin, and associated proteins form a periodic cytoskeletal structure in axons. *Science,* 339, 452-456. doi: 10.1126/ science.1232251.

[10] Sengupta, P., Jovanovic-Talisman, T., Skoko, D., Renz, M., Veatch, S., and Lippincott-Schwartz, J. (2011). Probing protein heterogeneity in the plasma membrane using PALM and pair correlation analysis. *Nature Methods,* 8, 969-975. doi: 10.1038/nmeth.1704.

[11] Renz, M., Daniels, B. R., Vámosi, G., Arias, I. M., and Lippincott-Schwartz, J. (2012). Plasticity of the asialoglycoprotein receptor deciphered by ensemble FRET imaging and single-molecule counting PALM imaging. *Proceedings of the National Academy of Sciences,* 109, 2989-2997. doi: 10.1073/pnas.1211753109.

[12] Das, S., Carnicer-Lombarte, A., Fawcett, J. W., and Bora, U. (2016). Bio-inspired nano tools for neuroscience. *Progress in Neurobiology*, 142, 1-22. doi: 10.1016/j.pn eurobio. 2016.04.008.

[13] Burnette, D., Manley, S., Sengupta, P., Sougrat, R., Davidson, M., Kachar, B., et al. (2011). A role for actin arcs in the leading edge advance of migrating cells. *Nature Cell Biology,* 13, 371-381. doi: 10.1038/ncb2205.

[14] Jaiswal, J. K., Goldman, E. R., Mattoussi, H., and Simon, S. M. (2004). Use of quantum dots for live cell imaging. *Nature Methods,* 1, 73-78. doi: 10.1038/nm eth1004-73.

[15] Kroto, H. W., Heath, J. R., O'Brien, S. C., Curl, R. F., and Smalley, R. E. (1985). C60: buckminsterfullerene. *Nature,* 318, 162-163. doi: 10.1038/3 18162a0.
[16] Iijima, S. (1991). Helical microtubules of graphitic carbon. *Nature,* 354, 56-58. doi: 10.1038/354056a0.
[17] Novoselov, K. S., Geim, A. K., Morozov, S. V., Jiang, D., Zhang, Y., Dubonos, S. V., et al. (2004). Electric field effect in atomically thin carbon films. *Science,* 306, 666-669. doi: 10.1126/science.1102896.
[18] Carvalho-de-Souza, J. L., Treger, J. S., Dang, B., Kent, S. B., Pepperberg, D. R., and Bezanilla, F. (2015). Photosensitivity of neurons enabled by cell-targeted gold nanoparticles. *Neuron,* 86, 207-217. doi: 10.1016/j.neuron.2 015.02.033.
[19] Orendorff R, Peck AJ, Zheng B, et al. (2017.) First in vivo traumatic brain injury imaging via magnetic particle imaging. *Physics in Medicine & Biology,* 62:3501-3509.
[20] Wong HL, Wu XY, Bendayan R. (2012). Nanotechnological advances for the delivery of CNS therapeutics. *Advanced Drug Delivery Reviews*, 64(7):686-700.
[21] Wong HL, Bendayan R, Rauth AM, Li Y, Wu XY. (2007). Chemotherapy with anticancer drugs encapsulated in solid lipid nanoparticles. *Advanced Drug Delivery Reviews*, 59(6):491-504.
[22] Dhawan S, Kapil R, Singh B. (2011). Formulation development and systematic optimization of solid lipid nanoparticles of quercetin for improved brain delivery. *Journal of Pharmacy and Pharmacology*, 63(3):342-351.
[23] Kuo YC, Liang CT. (2011). Inhibition of human brain malignant glioblastoma cells using carmustine-loaded catanionic solid lipid nanoparticles with surface anti-epithelial growth factor receptor. *Biomaterials*, 32(12):3340-3350.
[24] Ren, J., Shen, S., Wang, D., Xi, Z., Guo, L., Pang, Z., Qian, Y., Sun, X., & Jiang, X. (2012). The targeted delivery of anticancer drugs to brain glioma by PEGylated oxidized multi-walled carbon nanotubes modified with angiopep-2. *Biomaterials*, 33(11), 3324-3333. https://doi.org/10.1016/j.bio materials.2012.01.025.
[25] Fraczek-Szczypta, A. (2014). Carbon nanomaterials for nerve tissue stimulation and regeneration. *Materials Science and Engineering: C*, 34, 35-49.
[26] Matsumoto K, Shimizu N. (2013). Activation of the phospholipase C signaling pathway in nerve growth factor-treated neurons by carbon nanotubes. *Biomaterials*, 34(24):5988-5994.
[27] Aguilar ZP. (2013) Nanomedical Devices. *Nanomaterials for Medical Applications.* New York, New York: Elsevier; 2013. pp. 235-292.
[28] Tabatabaei SN. Towards MR-navigable nanorobotic carriers for drug delivery into the brain. In: *Robotics and Automation (ICRA).* IEEE International Conference, 2012, 14-18, May; Saint Paul, USA.
[29] Khalil ISM, Magdanz V, Sanchez S, Schmidt OG, Abelmann L, Misra S. Magnetic control of potential microrobotic drug delivery systems: nanoparticles, magnetotactic bacteria and self-propelled microjets. In: *Engineering in Medicine and Biology Society (EMBC).* 35th Annual International Conference of the IEEE; 2013, 3-7, July; Osaka, Japan.
[30] Martel S. Therapeutic bacterial nanorobots for targeted drug delivery deep inside tumors. in: *Nanorobotics.* New York, New York: Springer; 2013. pp. 323-329.

[31] Suter M, Zhang L, Siringil EC et al. (2013). Superparamagnetic microrobots: fabrication by two-photon polymerization and biocompatibility. *Biomedical Microdevices*, 15(6):997-1003.

[32] Hassan S, Ikram Ullah, Myeong Ok Kim, Jungwon Yoon. Neuro invasive multi-targeted drug delivery approach using swarm of nano-robotic carriers. In: *Intelligent Robotics and Applications*. Berlin Heidelberg: Springer; 2013. pp. 204-215.

[33] LaVan DA, McGuire T, Langer R. (2003). Small-scale systems for in vivo drug delivery. *Nature Biotechnology*, 21(10):1184-1191.

[34] Couvreur P, Vauthier C. (2006).Nanotechnology: intelligent design to treat complex disease. *Pharmaceutical Research*, 23(7):1417-1450.

[35] Ben-Yakar A, Bourgeois F. (2009). Ultrafast laser nanosurgery in microfluidics for genome-wide screenings. *Current Opinion in Biotechnology,* 20(1):100-105.

[36] Nguyen J, Ferdman J, Zhao M et al. (2011). Sub-surface, micrometer-scale incisions produced in rodent cortex using tightly-focused femtosecond laser pulses. *Lasers in Surgery and Medicine,* 43(5):382-391.

[37] Eversole DS (2013). *Plasmonic Laser Nanosurgery.* [online]. Available from: https://repositories.lib.utexas.edu/handle/2152/22244/.

[38] Hoy CL, Ferhanoglu O, Yildirim M et al. (2014). Clinical ultrafast laser surgery: recent advances and future directions. *IEEE Journal of Selected Topics in Quantum Electronics,* 20(2):242-255.

[39] Vogel A, Noack J, Hüttman G, Paltauf G. (2005). Mechanisms of femtosecond laser nanosurgery of cells and tissues. *Applied Physics*, 81(8):1015-1047.

[40] Jain K. Nanoneurology. In: *Applications of Biotechnology in Neurology*. New York, New York: Humana Press; 2013. pp. 563-574.

[41] Sheikh B, Raghed Atta, Mostafa Abdal Moneim. (2011). Chronic Brain cortical recording using siliconsubstrate microelectrode arrrays implanted in cerebral cortex International. *Journal of Academic Research*, 3(3):559-566.

[42] Qiao Y, Chen J, Guo X, Cantrell D, Ruoff R, Troy J. (2005). Fabrication of nanoelectrodes for neurophysiology:cathodic electrophoretic paint insulation and focused ion beam milling. *Nanotechnology*, 16(9):1598-1602.

[43] Kim W, Ng JK, Kunitake ME, Conklin BR, Yang P. (2007) Interfacing silicon nanowires with mammalian cells. *Journal of the American Chemical Society*, 29(23):7228-7229.

[44] Robinson JT, Marsela Jorgolli, Alex k. Shalek. (2012). Vertical nanowire electrode arrays as a scalable platform for intracellular interfacing to neuronal circuits. *Nature Nanotechnology*, 7(3):180-184.

[45] Ahmadi SA. Advanced planning and intra-operative validation for robot-assisted keyhole neurosurgery in ROBOCAST. In: *Advanced Robotics*. International Conference IEEE; 22-26 June 2009; Munich, Germany.

[46] De Momi E, Ferrigno G. (2010). Robotic and artificial intelligence for keyhole neurosurgery: the ROBOCAST project, a multi-modal autonomous path planner. *Proceedings of the Institution of Mechanical Engineers, Part H: Journal of Engineering in Medicine*, 224(5):715-727.

[47] Joskowicz L, Shohamb M, Shamira R, Freimana M, Zehavic E, Shoshan Y. Miniature robot-based precise targeting system for keyhole neurosurgery: concept

and preliminary results. In: *International Congress Series*; New York, New York, Elsevier; 2005, pp.618-623.

[48] Shoham M, Lieberman IH, Benzel EC. (2007). Robotic assisted spinal surgery-from concept to clinical practice. *Computer Aided Surgery*, 12(2):105-115.

[49] Shoham M, Lieberman IH, Benzel EC. (2007). Robotic assisted spinal surgery-from concept to clinical practice. *Computer Aided Surgery*, 12(2):105-115.

[50] Joskowicz L, Shamir R, Freiman M et al. (2006). Image-guided system with miniature robot for precise positioning and targeting in keyhole neurosurgery. *Computer Aided Surgery*, 11(4):181-193.

[51] Shamir, R, M Freiman, L Joskowicz, M Shoham, E Zehavi, Y Shoshan. (2005). Robot-assisted image-guided targeting for minimally invasive neurosurgery: intraoperative robot positioning and targeting experiment. *Medical Image Computing and Computer-Assisted Intervention,* 8 (2):131-138.

Chapter 10

Dental Care Associated with Patients Suffering from Neurological Disorders

Smriti Rastogi[1] and Radhika Rastogi[2,*]
[1]Medical Physiology, ICMR-SRF Department of Physiology,
King George's Medical University, Lucknow, Uttar Pradesh, India
[2]Saraswati Dental College, Lucknow, Uttar Pradesh, India

Abstract

A neurodegenerative disease can be defined as a progressive decline of the intellectual ability from a preceding level of performance (memory, space-time orientation, language, state of vigilance), involving inability in daily activities in a state of unimpaired consciousness. Commonly, we do not link oral manifestations with other parts of the body. But in reality, it has been surprisingly noted that various neurological disorders give rise to oral manifestations in an individual. A common reason for such link can be that since neurological diseases are much more prevalent in elderly people, therefore, they are more vulnerable to periodontal disease. Scientifically, neurological disorders interrupt the functioning of motor neurons which further causes an individual to perform basic oral functions such as, chewing, biting and swallowing. Generally, these symptoms are ignored but they lead to different dental diseases in future. Dental caries and periodontitis not only have effect on the dentition and tooth-supporting tissues, but also impact a number of systemic conditions. The loss of motor skills in neurological patients increases the risk for developing dental complications. Therefore, it is very important for people with neurological disorders to get proper dental care and regular check-ups to ensure oral health.

[*] Corresponding Author's Email: drradhika.rastogi@gmail.com.

In: New Perspectives in Neuroscience
Editors: Prachi Srivastava, Neha Srivastava and Prekshi Garg
ISBN: 978-1-68507-754-9

Keywords: neurological disorders, oral health, dental care, neurodegeneration

Introduction

In today's day and age it is imperative to stress upon and define the dental care that needs to be provided to patients with neurological disorders. There are a large number of neurological disorders that affect human beings, a lot of them affect the oral cavity directly, even those disorders that do not have a direct effect do affect the patient's overall mental health and have a deleterious impact on the upkeep of dental hygiene, status of the oral cavity, self-esteem and even the overall nutritional status of the patient. The contribution of non-communicable neurological disorders to total DALYs (disability adjusted life-years) in India doubled from 4,0% in 1990 to 8,2% in 2019. These neurological disorders include non-communicable neurological disorders (stroke, headache disorders, epilepsy, cerebral palsy, Alzheimer's disease and other dementias, brain and central nervous system cancer, Parkinson's disease, multiple sclerosis, motor neuron diseases, and other neurological disorders), communicable neurological disorders (encephalitis, meningitis, and tetanus), and injury-related neurological disorders (traumatic brain injuries and spinal cord injuries). Neurological disorders contribute 10% of the total disease burden in India [1]. Neurodegenerative disorders are some of the most challenging, devastating illnesses in medicine.

The central nervous system (CNS) and oral cavity have a close anatomical location. They have common vascular supply and a related embryological origin [2].

Seizures and Epilepsy

According to the International League Against Epilepsy, epilepsy is diagnosed when a person has 2 or more unprovoked seizures. It can be partial or generalized. It can be symptomatic, idiopathic or cryptogenic [3]. Patients who suffer from epilepsy, have poor oral health and dental status (greater number of decayed and missing teeth, have significantly fewer restored and replaced teeth, their degree of abrasion and periodontal indexes) is significantly worse than age-matched groups in the general (nonepileptic) population [4, 5].

Trauma

Generalized tonic–clonic seizures often cause oral injuries like tongue biting [6], tooth injuries [7] and even maxillofacial trauma [8]. Patients affected with epilepsy could be at an increased incidence of fracture because of the effect of drugs like benzodiazepines, antidepressants, antipsychotics, and enzyme-inducing antiepileptic drugs (e.g., phenytoin, phenobarbital, carbamazepine) which change the metabolism and renal clearance of vitamin D and can lead to osteopenia and osteomalacia [9]. Taking plenty of calcium and vitamin D supplementation (at least 1,000 mg and 400 IU daily, respectively) especially in patients consuming phenobarbital, phenytoin or primidone is vital [10].

Periodontal Problems

Approximately, 50% of patients on phenytoin are affected with gingival hyperplasia within 1 to 2 years of initiation of treatment. Regular use of either chlorhexidine or folic acid rinses or both, is recommended. Surgical reduction may be needed in severe cases [11]. Xerostomia and stomatitis are some effects of carbamazepine. Use of Valproic acid can cause direct bone marrow suppression, causing impaired wound healing and increased incidence of post-operative bleeding and infections. Thrombocytopenia is the commonest and best-known hematologic side effect of valproic acid; with the rate of occurrence varying from 5% to 40. In case of an elective surgery, certain investigations like bleeding time, fibrinogen level, prothrombin time, partial thromboplastin time and von Willebrand factor level — are required to assess the chance of peri- and postoperative bleeding [12].

Prosthodontic Problems

Patients suffering from epilepsy have chances of becoming edentulous earlier as compared to age matched controls [13]. Avoiding of incisal restorations, use of fixed rather than removable prostheses and inclusion of additional abutments if fixed partial dentures are used, using metal base for complete dentures and telescopic retention with denture bases made of metal or reinforced with metal for nearly edentulous patients is recommended for those with frequent partial seizures or generalized seizures concerned with falls and tonic–clonic. Cast gold fixed bridges or implant restorations are ideal for use in epileptic patients. All porcelain/ceramic restorations present a high risk of fracture, and removable prostheses run a greater risk of displacement causing aspiration pneumonia and should be avoided [14].

Dermatologic Problems

Appearance of rashes have been reported in of patients on phenytoin (around 5% to 7% patients) and patients using carbamazepine (around 5% to 17% patients) [15]. Toxic epidermal necrolysis (TEN) and Stevens–Johnson syndrome have also been reported [16].

Drug Interactions

Antifungal agents (fluconazole), metronidazole, and antibiotics (erythromycin) may affect the metabolism of certain antiepileptic drugs [17]. The combined administration of phenytoin and fluconazole is concerned with a significant rise in concentration of phenytoin in plasma, and dose of the latter may need changes to maintain concentrations of the therapeutic that are safe. Clarithromycin increases the plasma concentration of carbamazepine, and coadministration of these drugs should be observed closely to avoid carbamazepine toxicity [18]. Aspirin may displace valproic acid from plasma proteins and high doses of aspirin may inhibit metabolic pathways resulting in free serum valproate concentrations leading to subsequent toxicity [19].

Several disorders can often be mistaken for an epileptic seizure and the dentist must be careful to obtain a complete medical history along with the current medications and general health status of the patient [20].

Commonly confused conditions with epilepsy are:

- Hyperventilation
- Hypoglycaemia
- Migraine
- Transient ischemic attacks
- Syncope
- Pseudo seizure
- Transient global amnesia
- Sleep disorders

Dental Management of an Epileptic Patient

An in-depth knowledge of the patient's medical history and his/her current health status is a major requirement for treatment. Information regarding the type of epilepsy, frequency and duration of the last seizure should be known. Any stigma regarding epilepsy may prevent the patient from divulging the true status of the disease, careful and empathetic counselling may be required in such cases.

Certain questions may help to determine the health status of the patient. These include:

- Since when do you have epilepsy?
- What is the type and frequency of your seizures?
- What type of medication (if any) do you take?
- How do your seizures begin?
- Can you talk/respond appropriately during a seizure?
- Do you get confused/delirious/nauseous/tired after a seizure?
- When did your last seizure occur?

Certain important questions need to be asked on the day of the appointment:

- Have you had your seizure medication before coming to the clinic and have you been taking the medication regularly for the past few days?
- Have you had any over the counter drugs/alcohol today?
- Are you tired or do you feel unusually stressed today?
- Have you had any recent illness or seizures?

Preparations required while treating epileptic patients:

- List and study the medications currently taken by the patient. Know their effects, side effects, drug interactions and possible oral effects.
- Ascertain the frequency of dental appointments, take sufficient time after the dental procedure to give instructions regarding do's and do not's to the patients.

- Ensure that there is no direct light on the patient's eyes. Dark or colored glasses can be used as eye protection and the operating light must be controlled.
- Ensure medications for epilepsy have been taken properly.
- Accurate periodontal and surgical treatment of gingival hyperplasia to minimize damage to teeth and supporting structures and to maintain proper aesthetics.
- Treatment plan should be so designed so that there is minimun1risk of damaging/displacing restorations or prosthesis during the epileptic seizure.

Important point to note while treating patients suffering from epilepsy is the treatment of gingival hyperplasia and rectifying problems that have occurred in the oral cavity as a result of seizure trauma. The dentist should invest extra time in counselling the patient regarding the oral hygiene, he/she must tell the patient how vital dental health is for their overall well-being, must emphasize the importance of good nutrition on their systemic and gingival health. The importance of using a suitable dentifrice and any additional fluoride formulation to prevent decay of teeth must also be told especially to patients that are suffering from xerostomia. Frequent recall is recommended. Communication regarding dental techniques like explaining dental procedures beforehand and offering support and comfort during the treatment is always useful. Patients whose seizure activity does not respond to anticonvulsants may have to have a consultation with a neurologist prior to a dental appointment and require additional anticonvulsant or sedative medication. In some situations, use of conscious sedation and general anaesthesia, nitrous oxide or intravenous sedation may be necessary to safely and effectively provide dental care.

Seizure Management in Dental Clinic

Patient is in the clinic on the dental chair and at that time if seizure occurs:

- Remove all foreign material from the patient's mouth, move all dental instruments away from the patient, loosen his/her clothes.
- Adjust the dental chair of the patient so as to give proper support to the patient, place the patient in a supine position close to the floor.
- Assist the position on their lateral side to decrease the opportunity of regurgitation of materials or secretions in the patient's mouth.

- Do not aggressively stop the patient. Use only passive restraint to prevent the injury that may occur by the patient hitting nearby objects or to prevent them from falling off the chair.
- Do not take your hand close to the patient's mouth.
- Monitor the time of the seizures.
- Administration of the oxygen should be done at a rate of 6-8 L/min.
- If any of the conditions listed below occur, call for assistance immediately:
  - Duration of seizures is greater than 3 minutes.
  - If the patient has cyanosis from the very start of the seizure.

When the seizure subsides:

- Do not resume any dental treatment on that day.
- In the post-ictal phase, one should assess the level or consciousness of the patient by asking basic questions.
- Do not attempt to overtly restrict the patient, as this could confuse him or her.
- The patient should not leave the office in a delirious state or without someone to assist them, let him/her wait in the clinic until help or someone known to the patient arrives.
- Intimate the patient' family, in case the patient is all alone.
- Check the oral cavity for any injuries that might have occurred.
- In the post-ictal state, let the patient go home only with a responsible person (never send the patient back unassisted) to either his or her family physician or to the hospital.
- Call for emergency medical help if :
  1. Breathing difficulties occur post the seizure.
  2. Confusion, delirium, unconsciousness persists for more than 5 minutes post seizure.
  3. Injuries sustained during seizure.

Parkinson's Disease

The orofacial manifestations of Parkinson's disease are due to motor and sensory deficits and have a diverse spectrum of symptoms like:

Dysphagia

Is very common, [21] even normal swallowing of food or water can be a struggle for patients with Parkinson's disease. As the disease advances, there is increased risk of "silent aspiration" which leads to aspiration of minute amounts of food or saliva without normal protective reflexive mechanisms leading to a high prevalence of pneumonia [22].

Salivary Dysfunction

Patients may suffer from the various stages of decreasing saliva production or xerostomia on one hand and increased saliva production or sialorrhea as the normal saliva production is disturbed in Parkinson's disease. All the normal functions of saliva like lubrication, making food soluble, acting as buffer, normalizing the pH, enzymatic ability etc. are reduced or erratic, protection of teeth is compromised. Xerostomia exacerbates the rate of dental decay, especially roots caries and tooth sensitivity. Xerostomia may result from the disease process, or from drug therapy side effects (especially anti-cholinergic drugs), or from aging. Up to 78% of patients report Sialorrhea which may cause drooling with a high incidence of fungal infection (angular cheilitis) [23].

Burning Mouth

Burning mouth is common, compounded by xerostomia, medications, nutritional deficiencies, and even poor oral hygiene resulting from reduced muscle co-ordination required to grip a normal toothbrush. Halitosis is a chief complaint in most cases [21].

Changes in Taste and Smell

Patients are more vulnerable to changes in their taste and olfactory functions. Muscles in the gastrointestinal tract can also be affected resulting in heartburn or gastroesophageal reflux disease (GERD). Patients may complain of reduced flavour from food or, often, a bad taste in the mouth [21].

Other commonly associated symptoms are:

- Speech impairment.
- Soft voice
- Slurred words
- Fast speech
- Hesitation before speaking
- Mastication disorders Bruxism
- Subjective taste impairment

Difficulty in understanding the patient may result in reduced appreciation and reporting of pain or discomfort by the dental provider. It may be the first non- motor symptom that can indicate possible Parkinson's disease.

Bowel Dysfunction

Reduced control over bowel and bladder is a significant factor in planning dental treatment in patients of Parkinson's disease, especially while making elaborate treatment plans such as multiple crowns or implants.

Orthostatic Hypotension

Is frequently encountered in Parkinson's disease, and its diagnosis remains manometric (a fall of at least 20 and/or 10 mmHg in standing blood pressure) [16]. This is of special consideration when planning a dental procedure where the patient will be in a supine position for a long period of time [24].

Fatigue

Physical and mental fatigue ranges from a patient complaining of being tired or feeling uneasy in the middle of treatment to frequent requests to stop the procedure before it has been completed [21].

Anxiety

Young onset PD patients were more likely to experience frequent and severe anxiety than the late onset subjects. Mood swings and compulsive behaviour is common. This should be taken into consideration keeping in mind the safety of everyone.

Dental Management

A chronic progressive condition like Parkinson's disease results in varying degrees of increasing disability in important areas of activity like motor function, balance, mood condition, behaviour, activities related and essential to daily living and overall quality of life. Dyskinesia/ bradykinesia, loss of muscle tone, rigidity of the hands or/and face are often associated with a failure to maintain proper oral hygiene and results in recurrent infections of gums and periodontal tissue [25].

With the progressing tremors and poor muscle coordination, patients may face concerns with their grip and therefore overall dexterity to clean the teeth ranging from reduced grip over the toothbrush to squeezing toothpaste out of the tube. Toothbrushes with wider grip or power toothbrushes should be recommended and innovative solutions like fixing the brush inside bike handlebar grips or tennis balls so as to increase its surface area should be demonstrated to the patients to aid in maintenance of oral hygiene. Use of toothbrushes with softer bristles and smaller heads, mouthwashes, toothpaste pumps regular use of dental floss with holders (if possible), interproximal brushes all must be recommended and demonstrated to the patient so that he/she can choose the ideal method for maintaining oral hygiene.

Patients with reduced oral muscle control can be trained to either dip their brushes in the mouthwashes before brushing or to bend down over the sink and rinse, as gravity will allow the mouthwash to flow down the sink, thus reducing the incidence of uncontrolled swallowing by the patient. Patients having memory issues and difficulty remembering details about brushing or flossing can post sticky notes at the brushing area to remind them to follow the steps every day. Family members or caretakers can remind patients to brush and floss as well. Another strategy advocated for Parkinson's Disease patients is "one-handed preventive strategies," which allows them to use the stronger side of the body more often.

Table 1. Techniques for managing patients with Parkinson's disease in the dental environment

1.	Obtain and update a complete medical history • Ensure that medical history is up to date and prescriptions are updated regularly • Avoid drug interactions and note the progression of the disease through changes or additions to the medications list • Be familiar with the cardinal signs and symptoms of Parkinson's disease along with oral manifestations (xerostomia, dysphagia, etc.)
2.	Consult with the patient and his/her neurologist before treatment to determine the stage of Parkinson's disease • In later stages of the disease, patients may need to be referred to a hospital dental clinic for treatment
3.	Be aware of potential informed-consent issues • Discuss treatment needs with the patient, family members and/or caregivers who have power of attorney
4.	Preventive oral hygiene is integral • Patient, family members and/or caregivers should be instructed on proper oral hygiene techniques for their loved ones • Emphasize the importance of good oral care • Recommend that family or a friend accompany the patient to dental visits to ensure clear communication
5.	Dental visits should be short and scheduled in the morning • Coordinate appointments with the patient's medication schedule, if possible, to avoid manifestations of motor symptoms during dental procedures to avoid aspiration and potential for iatrogenic damage
6.	Be mindful of the potential for orthostatic hypotension • Patients may require assistance to be seated in the dental chair Patients should be raised slowly after completion of the procedure to prevent orthostatic hypotension • Orthostatic hypotension is mainly a symptom of anti-Parkinson's disease medications and should be prevented to avoid a medical emergency
7.	Consider sedation for complex procedures • Sedation may ensure patient comfort and facilitate efficiency of the dental practitioner • Patients should not surpass the state of minimal conscious sedation to avoid respiratory distress
8.	Avoid the use of cavitrons and piezo scalers • Magnetic devices may lead to transcranial stimulation and are therefore contraindicated in patients with Parkinson's disease.
9.	Be cautious when handling small items and consider the potential for aspiration • Consider fixed prostheses such as implants or fixed partial dentures • Use extreme caution during insertion of fixed partial dentures • Always place a rubber dam for restorative procedures • Review cardiopulmonary resuscitation protocols and be prepared to act accordingly in the case of an emergency

Dementia and Alzheimer's Disease

Alzheimer's disease can occur in three different stages: preclinical, mild cognitive impairment, and Alzheimer's disease dementia [27]. Patients' cognition can decrease in various spheres like memory, language, attention and executive function [28]. If the elderly patient has any of the following symptoms like impaired memory, reasoning, visuospatial ability, language function, for new information, or changes in personality or behaviours, then those individuals will be tested for diagnosis of dementia [29]. Alzheimer's disease is an incurable and progressive disorder that gets worsen with time [30]. Dental conditions aggregate due to improper self-care, polypharmacy, frailty, malnutrition, co-existing morbidity, dysphasia, xerostomia, dysphagia, the risk of aspiration pneumonia, and impaired cognition [31, 32, 33, 34]. Higher incidents of oral hygiene issues, gingival bleeding, periodontitis, and attachment loss, coronal and root caries, retained roots and plausible causes of orofacial pain, xerostomia and oral lesions, such as stomatitis and Candidiasis are observed in the patients suffering from dementia.

Elderly people with Alzheimer's disease can have low unstimulated and stimulated salivary flow rate of submandibular region [35]. Xerostomia is a primary factor for accentuating accumulation of plaque, halitosis, periodontal inflammation, candidiasis, caries rate, and an uncomfortable denture fit, thus forming a cycle of oral health that will undoubtedly impact the quality of life of an elderly individual [36].

Tooth loss leads to impaired masticatory manoeuvre which influences nutritional intake and may sometimes cause decreased cerebral stimulation and reduced flow of blood; thus, favouring the development or worsening of dementia [37]. A bidirectional association may exist between Alzheimer's and periodontal disease where both the diseases increase the effect of each other [38]. Aspiration pneumonia may emerge because of factors like age and frailty, diminished cough reflex, dysphagia, immunosuppression, sedatives, anti-depressants, impaired cognition, xerostomia, decreased salivary clearance, and inadequate oral hygiene [39, 40].

Treatment Planning

A few models are aimed at assisting in formulating the most appropriate management for individual cases. Examples of these models include:

- *OSCAR Five-Point Geriatric Dental Assessment:* There are five key areas involved in the planning of management of oral health for old people: oral (oral cavity), systemic (health history), capability (for self-care), autonomy (consent to care) and reality (financial, life expectancy, end-of-life care, etc.)
- *Seattle Care Pathway*: It aids dentists in evaluating functional statuses of patients' along with the possible risks to their oral health, and then develop oral health plans
- *SOAP (Subjective findings, Objective findings, Assessment and Plan)* [41, 42]: It is a documentation method that is used to record information of patients in a well organised manner [42]

As early detection depends on communication, but it is the parameter which is most affected in patients suffering from dementia or Alzheimer's. The key to planning, executing the dental treatment as well as sustaining the oral hygiene depends on an open and free interaction between the dentist, the caregiver of the patient and the patient himself. Building a rapport with the patient and gaining their trust is extremely crucial. The non- verbal communication is vital in establishing a good relationship with the patient as they can commonly misinterpret our actions. Dementia patients should be treated with a lot of patience and they should be instructed to follow only one command at a time, as they process commands slowly and have a lot of difficulty in following complex instructions. Therefore, while communicating with them instructions like sitting down, leaning back and asking them to open their mouths should be given step wise allowing them time to process the commands. We should concentrate on both non-verbal and verbal communication, gentle, pacifying words and empathetic communication and eye contact are vital so that the people are reassured as well as comfortable [43]. Elderly people usually have concomitant medical case, because of which they may take some specific medicines. All the appointments with the doctor should be short and crisp to ensure and understand low tolerance levels of elderly patients. The tell-show-do technique may aid in delivery of treatment. Treating the patient in the semi-supine position and the use of mouth props may help in providing comfort and safety to the patients [44]. A thorough examination, followed by routine recall examinations, as well as preventive and restorative care is essential. Prevention dental care from the time of diagnosis is the best care of all for these patients. The role of the caregiver cannot be overemphasized in this case, the dentist needs to involve the caregiver completely as scheduling of appointments, treatment protocol, compliance and adherence to the treatment of the patient depends as much on the caregiver as it does on the patient himself.

Stroke

This is a severe neurological condition caused by a sudden interruption or decrease of the cerebral blood flow, due to one or more pathological processes involving the cervical and/or the cerebral skull blood vessels, and is considered to be a serious neurological and/or neurosurgical emergency, which imposes a prompt and effective response [45-47].

The stroke is often fatal; if not fatal, it can determine several disabilities, more or less serious: speech deficiency, hemiplegia or paresis, different forms of paralysis or palsy with diminished or lost sensorial capacity and/or motor deficiency.

Important concerns while doing the dental management in ischemic stroke patients:

1. The risk of dental treatment upon a patient suffering from cerebrovascular ischemic disease and the fact that
2. Lesions of the oral cavity that can be induced by ischemia of the carotidian afferent branches [48, 49].

Myasthenia Gravis

Causes generalized muscle weakness, including the muscles of the face, tongue, and neck, patients may hold their jaws in a slack position with the mouth open. The problem worsens towards the end of the day and with fatigue or stress [50, 51, 52, 53, 54].

Dental Considerations

Dental treatment should be scheduled at a time when the patient is not fatigued, and preferably during remission of the disease. Appointments need to be made 1-2 hours after the patient has taken his or her medication (an anticholinesterase, e.g., pyridostigmine), preferably in the morning.

Table 2. Dental management of patients with stroke

1.	• Short, stress-free appointments scheduled in the morning.
2.	• Disabled patients should be helped by the nurse to sit on dental chair, their airways should be free and they should be accompanied by the persons taking care of them, especially if speech difficulties are present
3.	• Dentist should stand in front of the patient, without mask, should look him in the eyes, should move slowly and questions should be simple and clear, for direct answers (yes/no)
4.	• Anamnesis should be simple relevant showing patient's risk factors. If the medical record shows high blood pressure, cardiac diseases, transient vascular accidents, diabetes, dyslipidaemia, coronary atherosclerosis, (heavy) smoking, old age, then such a patient is prone to stroke and/or myocardial infarction
5.	• History of past strokes needs to be elicited: date, seriousness, treatment, disabilities.
6.	• The dentist may encounter situations when patient's speech has not yet been affected, but the patient is unaware of the extent of palsy or situations when a patient with brain injury on his right side is neglecting his left side of the body
7.	• Blood pressure and pain should be monitored and under control during the entire intervention.
8.	• Emergency dental treatment is allowed six months after stroke, it should be performed carefully, by neurologist's advice and some precautions are needed, according to the specific characters of the stroke: • Anticoagulant drugs like heparin should be stopped at least 6-12 hours before treatment, if the dental treatment produces bleeding (teeth extraction, pulpectomy, subgingival scaling, periodontal surgery) as anticoagulant systemic medication may cause serious haemorrhage that could create problems in a clinical setting. • Six hours after bleeding, when blood clots are built up, heparin systemic treatment can be resumed. • If there is some other anticoagulant medication involved, it should be stopped several hours or days before bleeding dental treatment, only after determining the International Clotting Rate (ICR) and decision depends on neurologist's advice. • The dentist should be ready for emergency intervention in case of local haemorrhage, with haemostatic medication and cautery, blood pressure should be monitored and oxygen therapy device is needed in dental office. • The minimal amount of anaesthetic solutions should be injected, concentration of added epinephrine should be very low (1:100.000 or 1:200.000). • Use of gingival retraction cord soaked with epinephrine should be avoided. • Metronidazole and tetracycline should be avoided, since they may affect blood clotting.

Table 2. (Continued)

9.	• If symptoms of stroke occur in the dental clinic, then patient should get oxygen therapy immediately and referral to hospital should be done immediately.
10.	• Patients with transient ischemic attack (TIA) or with stroke in their medical record have a very complex dental and periodontal pathology.
11.	• Poor oral hygiene is common in patients with physical disabilities. Use of electric toothbrushes, dental floss, oral irrigation and prophylaxis using chlorhexydine and fluoride is recommended.
12.	• Patients with speech and deglutition disabilities due to paralysis of orofacial muscles, with loss of sensitivity of the tissues, with flaccid, multiple pleated and asymmetrically positioned tongue, with dysphagia, may present accumulation of food residues on teeth, tongue, oral mucosa. They must learn to clean their teeth and oral cavity using only one hand or to get/accept another person's help, in order to avoid caries, periodontitis, halitosis or oral mucosa diseases.
13.	• Edentulous patients are advised to get fixed prosthodontic treatment, because of the difficulties of insertion and removal of removable dentures.
14.	• Poor oral care after a stroke can have serious physical, psychological and social consequences and adversely affect quality of life.
15.	• Aspiration pneumonia: Has the highest attributable mortality in stroke patients • Dysphagia and loss of sensation • Stasis of saliva and food in the oral cavity is commonly seen • Reduced tongue pressure and altered lateral movements result in denture wearing and retention problems and stomatitis. • Oral discomfort and pain, oral infections (especially oral candidiasis) are common • Eating, drinking and tooth brushing can be severely disrupted • High carriage of and colonisation by aerobic Gram-negative bacteria has been observed in stroke patients.

Anxious patients may benefit from a low dose of an anxiolytic benzodiazepine such as such as diazepam (Valium) or lorazepam (Ativan) taken prior to treatment. Procaine anaesthetics should not be used for local anaesthesia.

In the patient with a dental abscess, only the antibiotics penicillin or erythromycin can be safely used to treat infection. Drugs to be avoided include the tetracyclines, clindamycin, lincomycin, sulphonamides, and aminoglycosides. For pain, paracetamol coupled with a narcotic (e.g., codeine) may be helpful. Aspirin has been associated with cholinergic crisis in patients taking anticholinesterases, so it should be avoided. Since patients with myasthenia gravis often have impaired respiration, special consideration needs to be taken for maintaining oxygenation during procedures involving conscious sedation. In fact, it is best to treat these patients in an inpatient hospital setting. The drugs often used in conscious sedation (e.g., opioids, barbiturates) may potentiate or aggravate breathing difficulty in myasthenia gravis patients [55].

Facial Paralysis

Through the cranial nerves, most of the motor and sensory organs in the orofacial region have a connection with the CNS [56, 57]. The disorders can mainly be divided into various groups based on their aetiology such as the neoplasia of neural origin, diseases of cranial nerves, and neurological disorders by its orofacial manifestations [58]. Cranial nerve V, VII, IX, X, and XII disorders are important for a dentist because all sensory and motor functions in the orofacial region are under the control of these nerves. Bell's palsy, trigeminal neuralgia, vago-glossopharyngeal neuralgia, sphenopalatine neuralgia, post-herpetic neuralgia, atypical facial pain, hypoglossal nerve paralysis, and auriculotemporal syndrome are among common cranial nerve disorders [59-61]. Conditions causing loss of function of the seventh cranial nerve include multiple sclerosis, infection (e.g., syphilis, HIV disease, Lyme disease, leprosy), sarcoidosis, cholesteatoma, Bell palsy, and several intracranial problems (e.g., tumour, trauma). Upper and lower motor neuron abnormality can be differentiated by the resulting loss of function. Many of these conditions affect oral health [62, 63, 64, 65, 66, 67].

Dental Considerations

Loss of taste can occur and is associated with abnormality of the chorda tympani.

In cases involving Bell palsy, the corneas should be protected during dental treatment. In other cases of facial palsy, there may be accumulation of food debris, potentially increasing dental plaque. Patients should be instructed in techniques to be used after eating aimed at eliminating the material. Leaking of saliva at the corners of the mouth may predispose the patient to angular cheilitis. An antifungal cream appropriately placed may be useful if fungal infection emerges.

Placement of a splint may be helpful in improving facial aesthetics. Other approaches may include appliances anchored to the teeth. Suturing may also be useful. Pain in the region of the ear/temporomandibular joint may be the result of inflammation of the geniculate ganglia of the facial nerve. Avoidance of misdiagnosis (temporomandibular joint pathology) is important. Facial dyskinesias can lead to tongue or jaw movement that can confound dental treatment. Bruxism can lead to tooth wear or fracture. Patients with facial dyskinesias may benefit from predental treatment prescription of a benzodiazepine. Sensory deficits associated with conditions involving the fifth cranial nerve may be the result of conditions such as Paget disease or peripheral lesions involving the bones and the canals. Brain stem lesions can affect mastication and cause mouth-opening difficulty. Facial paralysis can result from alveolar nerve blocks and in some cases, this can be permanent [55].

Conclusion

Dentists faced with patients affected by one of these disorders are confronted with the major problems of cognition, mobility, and behaviour, as well as of dental maintenance. While treatment of patients with progressive neurodegeneration remains daunting, increased knowledge of the aetiology and pathogenesis of these diseases has provided new opportunities and a new understanding of their treatment needs. Given the far-reaching impact of neurological disorders and the vast proportion of the population that suffers from them, it is high time that a detailed dental regime for prophylaxis, maintenance and complete care of patients suffering from neurological disorders be planned and implemented. The dentist is at a tricky position here as some disorders like epilepsy lead to flattening of occlusal surfaces of teeth on account of clenching, palsies can commonly cause drooling of saliva and on the other hand medications given in the treatment of these disorders result in xerostomia. There must be customization of dental care when treating a patient with neurological disorder so that he gets the best care especially designed to treat and as far as possible slow down the harmful effect of his or her disorder on the overall dental health. The aim of the dentist should be to provide the best possible dental care keeping in mind the long-term effects of both the disorder and the medication given to treat it.

References

[1] Gagandeep Singh, Meenakshi Sharma, G Anil Kumar, N Girish Rao, Kameshwar Prasad et al. The burden of neurological disorders across the states of India: the global burden of disease study 1990–2019. *Lancet Global Health* 2021; 9: e1129–44 https://doi.org/10.1016/ S2214-109X(21) 00164.

[2] Kirtana Gopalasamy, V. Vishnu Priya, R. Gayathri. Knowledge and awareness of neurological disorders among dental students. *Drug Intervention Today* 2019; 11(12).

[3] Proposal for revised classification of epilepsies and epileptic syndromes. Commission on Classification and Terminology of the International League Against Epilepsy. *Epilepsia* 1989; 30(4):389–99.

[4] Karolyhazy K, Kovacs E, Kivovics P, Fejerdy P, Aranyi Z. Dental status and oral health of patients with epilepsy: an epidemiologic study. *Epilepsia* 2003; 44(8):1103–8.

[5] Karolyhazy K, Kivovics P, Fejerdy P, Aranyi Z. Prosthodontic status and recommended care of patients with epilepsy. *Journal of Prosthetic Dentistry* 2005; 93(2):177–82.

[6] Pick L, Bauer J. Zahnmedizin und epilepsie [*Dentistry and epilepsy*]. *Der Nervenarzt* 2001; 72(12):946–9.

[7] Buck D, Baker GA, Jacoby A, Smith D, Chadwick DW. Patients' experiences of injury as a result of epilepsy. *Epilepsia* 1997; 38(4):439–44.

[8] Aragon CE, Burneo JG, Helman J. Occult maxillofacial trauma in epilepsy. *Journal of Contemporary Dental Practice* 2001; 2(4):26–32.

[9] Mattson RH, Gidal BE. Fractures, epilepsy, and antiepileptic drugs. *Epilepsy Behavior* 2004; 5(Suppl 2):S36–40.

[10] Sato Y, Kondo I, Ishida S, Motooka H, Takayama K, Tomita Y, and others. Decreased bone mass and increased bone turnover with valproate therapy in adults with epilepsy. *Neurology* 2001; 57(3):445–9.

[11] Stoopler ET, Sollecito TP, Greenberg MS. Seizure disorders: update of medical and dental considerations. *General Dentistry* 2003; 51(4):361–6.

[12] Archarya S, Bussel JB. Hematologic toxicity of sodium valproate. *Pediatric Hematology and Oncology* 2000; 22(1):62–5.

[13] Karolyhazy K, Kivovics P, Fejerdy P, Aranyi Z. Prosthodontic status and recommended care of patients with epilepsy. *Journal of Prosthetic Dentistry* 2005; 93(2):177–82.

[14] Karolyhazy K, Kovacs E, Kivovics P, Fejerdy P, Aranyi Z. Dental status and oral health of patients with epilepsy: an epidemiologic study. *Epilepsia* 2003; 44(8):1103–8.

[15] Hirsch LJ, Weintraub DB, Buchsbaum R, Spencer HT, Straka T, Hager M, and other. Predictors of lamotrigine-associated rash. *Epilepsia* 2006; 47(2):318–22.

[16] Mockenhaupt M, Messenheimer J, Tennisj P, Schlingmann J. Risk of Stevens-Johnson syndrome and toxic epidermal necrolysis in new users of antiepileptics. *Neurology* 2005; 64(7):1134–8.

[17] Goulden KJ, Dooley JM, Camfield PR, Fraser AD. Clinical valproate toxicity induced by acetylsalicylic acid. *Neurology* 1987; 37(8):1392–4.

[18] Patsalos PN, Frosher W, Pisani F, Van Rijn CM. The importance of drug interactions in epilepsy therapy. *Epilepsia* 2002; 43(4):365–85.

[19] Miners JO. Drug interactions involving aspirin (acetylsalicylic acid) and salicylic acid. *Clinical Pharmacokinet* 1989; 17(5):327–44.

[20] Peter L. Jacobse, Oleksandra Eden. Epilepsy and the dental management of the epileptic patient. *Journal of Contemporary Dental Practice,* 2008 ; 9(1) :54-62.

[21] Satbir Grover, Nelson Rhodus. Dental management of Parkinson's disease *Northwest Dentistry* 2011; 90(6):13-19 http://www.mndental.org/features/2011/12/01/357.

[22] Michaell A. Huber. Parkinson's disease and oral health. *The American Parkinson Disease Association, Educational Supplement #7,* 2007; 1-4.

[23] Friedlander AH. Sjögren syndrome. *Journal of the American Dental Association* 2009; 140(3):279.

[24] Kyle G. The physical, social and emotional effects of bowel dysfunction in Parkinson's disease. *Nurses Times* 2010; 106(33):20-2.

[25] Nakayama Y, Washio M, Mori M. (2004) Oral health conditions in patients with Parkinson's disease. *American Journal of Epidemiology* 2004; 14(5):143-50.

[26] M. S. Lee, P. Lam, and E. Ernst, "Effectiveness of tai chi for Parkinson's disease: a critical review," *Parkinsonism and Related Disorders* 2008; 14(8):589-594.

[27] Hane, FT, Robinson, M, Lee, BY, Bai, O, Leonenko, Z, Albert, MS. Recent progress in Alzheimer's disease research, part 3: diagnosis and treatment. *Journal of Alzheimers Disease*. 2017; 57: 645-665.

[28] Albert, MS, Dekosky, ST, Dickson, D, Dubois, B., Feldman, HH, Fox, NC, Gamst, A., Holtzman, DM, Jagust, WJ, Petersen, RC, et al. The diagnosis of mild cognitive impairment due to Alzheimer's disease: recommendations from the National Institute on Aging-Alzheimer's Association workgroups on diagnostic guidelines for Alzheimer's disease. *Alzheimers & Dementia Journal* 2011 ; 7: 270-279.

[29] McKhann, GM, Knopman, DS, Chertkow, H, Hyman, BT, Jack, CR, Kawas, CH, Klunk, WE, Koroshetz, WJ, Manly, JJ, Mayeux, R, et al. The diagnosis of dementia due to Alzheimer's disease: recommendations from the National Institute on Aging-

Alzheimer's Association workgroups on diagnostic guidelines for Alzheimer's disease. *Alzheimers & Dementia Journal* 2011 ; 7 : 263-269.
[30] Chavez, EM, Wong, LM, Subar, P., Young, DA, Wong, A. Dental care for geriatric and special needs populations. *Dental Clinics of North America.* 2018 ; 62 : 245-267.
[31] Henry, RG, Smith, BJ. Managing older patients who have neurologic disease: Alzheimer disease and cerebrovascular accident. *Dental Clinics of North America* 2009 ; 53: 269-294.
[32] Marchini, L, Ettinger, R, Caprio, T, Jucan, A. Oral health care for patients with Alzheimer's disease: an update. *Special Care in Dentistry* 2019 ; 39: 262-273.
[33] Chavez, EM, Wong, LM, Subar, P., Young, DA, Wong, A. Dental care for geriatric and special needs populations. *Dental Clinics of North America.* 2018 ; 62: 245-267.
[34] Huang, ST, Chiou, CC, Liu, HY. Risk factors of aspiration pneumonia related to improper oral hygiene behavior in community dysphagia persons with nasogastric tube feeding. *Journal of Dental Sciences.* 2017 ; 12: 375-381.
[35] Delwel, S, Binnekade, TT, Perez, RSGM, Hertogh, CMPM, Scherder, EJA, Lobbezoo, F. Oral hygiene and oral health in older people with dementia: a comprehensive review with focus on oral soft tissues. *Clinical Oral Investigations.* 2018 ; 22: 93-108.
[36] Turner, MD, Ship, JA. Dry mouth and its effects on the oral health of elderly people. *Journal of American Dentistry Association* 2007 ; 138: 15S-20S.
[37] Campos, CH, Ribeiro, GR, Garcia, RCMR. Mastication and oral health-related quality of life in removable denture wearers with Alzheimer disease. *Journal of Prosthetic Dentistry* 2018 ; 119: 764-768.
[38] Pazos, P, Leira, A, Dominguez, C, Pias-Peleteiro, JM, Blanco, J, Aldrey, JM. Association between periodontal disease and dementia: a literature review. *Neurologia* 2018 ; 33: 602-613.
[39] Cichero, JAY. Age-related changes to eating and swallowing impact frailty: Aspiration, choking risk, modified food texture and autonomy of choice. *Geriatrics* 2018 ; 3: 69.
[40] Taylor, GW, Loesche, WJ, Terpenning, MS. Impact of oral disease on systemic health in the elderly: Diabetes Mellitus and Aspiration Pneumonia. *Journal of Public Health Dentistry.* 2000 ; 60: 313-320.
[41] Chavez, EM, Wong, LM, Subar, P, Young, DA, Wong, A. Dental care for geriatric and special needs populations. *Dental Clinics of North America.* 2018 ; 62: 245-267.
[42] Oong, EM, An, GK. Treatment planning considerations in older adults. *Dental Clinics of North America.* 2014 ; 58: 739-755.
[43] Brennan, LJ, Strauss, J. Cognitive impairment in older adults and oral health considerations: Treatment and management. *Dental Clinics of North America* 2014 ; 58: 815-828.
[44] Robbins, MR. Neurologic diseases in special care patients. *Dental Clinics of North America* 2016 ; 60: 707-735.
[45] Brandt T, Orberk E, Weber R, et al. Pathogenesis of cervical arterial dissection. *Neurology* 2001; 57:24-30.

[46] Boccalon H. *Guide practique des maladies vasculaires*. [*Practical guide to vascular diseases*]. Paris, France: MMI Ed., 2001.

[47] Buhlin K, Gustafsson A, Pockley AG, et al. Risk factors for cardiovascular disease in patients with periodontitis. *European Heart Journal* 2003; 24:2099-107.

[48] Babes K, Popa AR, Babes A. Ateroscleroza si diabetul zaharat. [*Atherosclerosis and diabetes*]. *Revista Medicala Nationala* 1998; ii(1):43-9.

[49] Bodnar D, Popa BM, Bodnar T. Malformatii vasculare cervico-faciale. Consecinte neurologice în practica stomatologica. [Cervico-facial vascular malformations. Neurological consequences in dental practice]. *Sinteze si rezumate la a IV-a Conferinta Nationala de Stroke (AVC). Revista Romana de Stroke (AVC)* 3-5 Oct. 2001.

[50] Lotia S, Randall C, Dawson LJ, Longman Dental management of the myasthenic patient. *Dent Update* 2004; 4:237-42.

[51] Tolle L. Myasthenia gravis: a review for dental hygienists. *J Dent Hyg*. 2007 Winter. 81(1):12.

[52] Yarom N, Barnea E, Nissan J, Gorsky M. Dental management of patients with myasthenia gravis : a literature review. *Oral Surg Oral Med Oral Pathol Oral Radiol Endod*. 2005 ; 100 (2): 158-63.

[53] Patil PM, Singh G, Patil SP. Dentistry and the myasthenia gravis patient: a review of the current state of the art. *Oral Surg Oral Med Oral Pathol Oral Radiol*. 2012 ; 114(1):e1-8.

[54] Pregerson B. Myasthenia gravis in elderly man with slurred speech. *Patient Care Online*. [online]. Available from : https://www.patientcareonline.com/view/myasthenia-gravis-elderly-man-slurred-speech/. 2012.

[55] Burgess, Jeff. Management of the dental patient with neurological disease. *Medscape*. [online]. Available from : https://emedicine.medscape.com/article/2091727-overview2017/.

[56] Friedman MH. Atypical facial pain: The consistency of ipsilateral. Maxillary area tenderness and elevated temperature. *J Am Dent Assoc* 1995; 126:855-60.

[57] Fauci AS, Braunwald E, Isselbacher KJ, Wilson JD, Martin JB, Kasper DL, et al. *Harrison's Principles of Internal Medicine*. 14th ed. United States of America: McGraw-Hill Companies, Inc.; 1998. pp. 2307-451.

[58] Amanat D. Oral and maxillofacial manifestations of neurological diseases in southern provinces of Iran. *J Dent Shiraz Univ Med Sci* 2012;13:23-8.

[59] Wood NK, Goaz PW. *Differential Diagnosis of Oral and Maxillofacial Lesions*. 5th ed. St Louis, MO: Mosby-Year Book, Inc.; 1997. p. 329-33.

[60] Dev S. Oral manifestations of neurological disorders: a comprehensive overview. *Dent Hypotheses* 2014;5:78-9.

[61] Rushton B. Glossopharyngeal neuralgia. *Arch Neurol* 1982;38:201.

[62] Bagchi G, Nath DK. Restoration of facial symmetry in a patient with bell palsy using a modified maxillary complete denture: a case report. *Int J Prosthodont*. 2012; 25(3):290-3 (ISSN: 0893-2174).

[63] Pereira FP, Guskuma MH, Luvizuto ER, Faco EF, Magro-Filho O, Hochuli-Vieira E. Unilateral facial paralysis caused by Ramsay Hunt syndrome. *J Craniofac Surg*. 2011; 22(5):1961-3 (ISSN: 1536-3732).

[64] Selvi F, Guven E, Mutlu D Clinical management of microstomia due to the static treatment of facial paralysis and oral rehabilitation with dental implants. *J Craniofac Surg.* 2011; 22(3):967-9 (ISSN: 1536-3732).

[65] Chevalier V, Arbab-Chirani R, Tea SH, Roux M. Facial palsy after inferior alveolar nerve block: case report and review of the literature. *Int J Oral Maxillofac Surg.* 2010; 39(11):1139-42 (ISSN: 1399-0020).

[66] Sajjan MC, Krishna RG. Lip-support prosthesis--a unique approach in management of bilateral facial palsy. *Quintessence Int.* 2007; 38(8):e517-20 (ISSN: 1936-7163).

[67] Ilea A, Cristea A, Tărmure V, Trombitaş VE, Câmpian RS, Albu S. Management of patients with facial paralysis in the dental office: A brief review of the literature and case report. *Quintessence Int.* 2014; 45(1):75-86 (ISSN: 1936-7163).

Chapter 11

Current Trends in Oral Neurosciences

Apurva K. Srivastava*

Department of Microbiology,
Sardar Patel Post Graduate Institute of Dental and Medical Sciences,
Lucknow, India

Abstract

Neurosciences is a multidisciplinary science involving the scientific study of the nervous system. The central nervous system and oral cavity have a close anatomical relationship. The mouth and face are the location for 30-40% of the body's sensory and motor nerves. Neuroscience is relevant to oral and dental areas, as many neurally-based functions, such as pain, taste, chewing, swallowing and salivation, are manifested in the orofacial area and disorders of these functions are quite common. Some diseases related to central nervous system in the Oro- mandibular and Maxillofacial regions, diseases like oral neurological disorders, cognitive deficits in psychiatric patients, oromandibular movement disorder, and cognitive impairment that may be related to masticatory deficits gain a significant importance in this context. New studies in this field of neural pathways and the study of its functions along with its adaptability to pain injury, and healing have opened new vistas. The neurological related disturbances in the oral/dental/maxillofacial region can be:

Sensory disturbances - trigeminal neuralgia, glossopharyngeal neuralgia, persistent idiopathic facial pain, burning mouth syndrome, cluster headache.

Motor disturbances that are of importance in this area are – Bell's palsy, central poststroke pain, multiple sclerosis, syringobulbia, and Tourette syndrome.

---

* Corresponding Author's Email: dr.aksrivastav@gmail.com.

In: New Perspectives in Neuroscience
Editors: Prachi Srivastava, Neha Srivastava and Prekshi Garg
ISBN: 978-1-68507-754-9

Movement disorders - cerebral palsy and Parkinson disease.

Infections such as neurosyphilis, leprosy, and herpes zoster.

Some of the main neurological diseases and conditions which may affect the oral/dental/maxillofacial regions have been described in this chapter.

Introduction: Neurologic Disorders of the Maxillofacial Region

Neurosciences is a multidisciplinary science involving the scientific study of the nervous system. A thorough understanding of this concept from the peripheral neuromuscular to the central nervous systems is very much needed. The scientific advances and the increased interest in this field in recent years especially in biotechnology, molecular biology, genetics, is quite promising.

Neuroscience is relevant to oral and dental areas, as many nervous functions especially of taste, chewing, swallowing, pain and salivation, present themselves first in the oral, dental and maxillofacial areas [1]. New studies in this field of neural pathways and the study of its functions along with its adaptability to pain injury, and healing has opened new vistas. Neurological diseases of this Maxillofacial regions, cognitive deficits in psychiatric patients, mandibular jaw movement disorder, and cognitive defects that maybe related to masticatory impairment has gained considerable significance.

An understanding of the nerve supply of the Oral and facial region is necessary to understand the neurological disorders of the maxillofacial region.

Nerve Supply

The 12 pair of nerves which arise directly from brain are called cranial nerves and they are classified as given below.

I. Olfactory nerve
II. Optic nerve
III. Oculomotor nerve
IV. Trochlear nerve
V. Trigeminal nerve
VI. Abducens nerve
VII. Facial nerve

VIII. Vestibulocochlear nerve
IX. Glossopharyngeal nerve
X. Vagus nerve
XI. Accessory nerve
XII. Hypoglossal nerve

The nerve supply to the oral, dental and maxillofacial region is of three types:

- Sensory
- Motor
- Autonomic

The *main nerves of* the oral, dental and maxillofacial region are:

- *Trigeminal Nerve (V Cranial Nerve): Sensory and Motor*

  Trigeminal nerve contains both sensory and motor fibers. It is also the largest cranial nerve [1]. It has three terminal branches, - ophthalmic nerve (V1), maxillary nerve (V2), and mandibular nerve (V3) respectively. The mandibular division carries both sensory and motor fibers while ophthalmic and maxillary nerves are purely sensory. The maxillary nerve (V2) provides sensory supply to the middle third of the face. Its fibers also supply the lacrimal gland and mucous glands of the nasal mucosa. The trigeminal nerve supplies sensation to meninges, skin of anterior part of the head, nasal and oral cavities and the teeth. It also provides motor innervation to the muscles of mastication.
- *Facial Nerve (VII Cranial Nerve)*

  The facial nerve provides both sensory and motor functions, including moving muscles used for facial expressions and some muscles in the jaw providing a sense of taste for most of the tongue. It also supplies fibers to the glands in the head and neck area, such as salivary glands and lacrimal glands.
- *Glossopharyngeal Nerve (IX Cranial Nerve)*

  This nerve provides for the functions like sending sensory information from the sinuses, back of the throat, parts of the inner ear, and the posterior part of tongue. It also provides, stimulating voluntary movement of stylopharyngeus muscle at the back of the throat, helping in swallowing.

- *Hypoglossal Nerve (X Cranial Nerve)*

  As the name suggests this nerve is responsible for the movement of tongue muscles.

The identification and management of neurologic diseases and disorders is quite challenging and depends to a large extent on proper clinical, radiological and laboratory diagnosis and investigations. The anatomy of the maxillofacial region is quite complex and so are the related neurologic disorders. The neurological related disturbances in the oral/dental/ maxillofacial region can be:

- *Sensory disturbances* - trigeminal neuralgia, glossopharyngeal neuralgia, persistent idiopathic facial pain, burning mouth syndrome, cluster headache, geniculate neuralgia, and temporal arteritis.
- *Motor disturbances* that are of importance in this area are – Bell's palsy, central poststroke pain, multiple sclerosis, syringobulbia, and Tourette syndrome.
- *Movement disorders* - cerebral palsy and Parkinson disease, and their maxillofacial manifestations.
- *Infections* such as neurosyphilis, leprosy, and herpes zoster.

The diseases of nervous system have been extensively studied in various specialties of biomedical sciences like as otology, ophthalmology, neurology, neurosurgery, and dentistry. The central nervous system and oral cavity have a close anatomical relationship. The mouth and face are the location for 30-40% of the body's sensory and motor nerves. The nervous system comprises the brain, spinal cord, and spinal and peripheral nerves, functional capacity and life itself may be lost when disease or damage occurs. Some of the neurological diseases/conditions which may affect the oral/dental/maxillo-facial regions are described below.

Trigeminal Neuralgia (Tic Douloureux)

Trigeminal neuralgia (TN), also called *tic douloureux*, is a form of neuropathic pain, chronic in nature, due to the involvement of trigeminal or 5th cranial nerve. TN is a form of (pain associated with nerve injury or nerve lesion.) According to the International Classification of Headache Disorders, Third

Edition (ICHD-3), trigeminal neuralgia, is characterized by sudden onset of recurrent unilateral electric shock-like, stabbing, or shooting pain lasting between a fraction of a second and 2 minutes. It occurs along the anatomical distribution of the fifth cranial nerve, mainly affecting the maxillary (V2) and maxillary (V3) divisions of the trigeminal nerve and almost always exhibits a trigger zone, stimulation of which initiates paroxysm of pain [2.] The pain is often accompanied by a brief facial spasm or tic. The triggers of pain can be a simple facial touch, tooth brushing, shaving, eating, or even talking, or a blast of cold air. The sporadic episodes of pain sometimes terminate abruptly with intermittent painless periods giving the patient a false sense of relief.

Types of Trigeminal Neuralgia

1. Classic trigeminal neuralgia- Idiopathic (no evident disorder)/Classic (vascular compression of the nerve).
2. Secondary (symptomatic) trigeminal neuralgia: etiology ranges from injury, infections, brain tumors, multiple sclerosis, etc. Sometimes history of dental is also seen.

Women above 40 years of age are seen to be affected more with a prevalence of 0.07% to 0.3% [3].

The trigeminal neuralgia remains a mystery since many centuries. The cause of this disease process is unknown. It is usually idiopathic, but many reasons have been proposed like, pressure on the nerve by tumors or vascular anomalies. Abnormal vessels, aneurysms, tumors, chronic meningeal inflammation, or other lesions may irritate trigeminal nerve roots along the pons [4]. Various granulomatous and nongranulomatous infections involving the 5th cranial nerve can cause a similar pain. Patient reports with a history of excruciating shooting sharp pain sometimes like an electric shock usually on one side of the face. The pain is so severe that it compromises basic functions like talking or eating. Another set of symptoms reported by other patients include, constant burning pain, usually affecting one side of face, with right side of the face is affected in more patients than the left by a ratio of about 1.7:1 [5]. Initially the symptoms reported are mild but they gradually increase in severity as the time progresses. Later, the pain may be so severe there is constant fear of an attack of pain, and many sufferers have attempted suicide to put an end to their torment. The 'trigger zones,' which precipitate an attack when touched, are commonly seen on nose, lips, cheeks, and around the eyes.

Diagnosis of trigeminal neuralgia is made from a well-taken history. The classic clinical pattern will lead towards the diagnosis. Some supplementary investigations like MRI and CT scan may help to exclude an uncommon space occupying esion or aberrant vessel compression on the nerve roots. Medicinal treatment includes anticonvulsant drugs like Phenytoin, Carbamazepine. Injecting Long-acting anesthetic agents - without adrenaline such as bupivacaine (with or without corticosteroids), and alcohol (95% absolute alcohol) near the trigger zone to alleviate the symptoms have been suggested. Peripheral neurectomy sectioning of the nerve at the mental foramen, or at the supraorbital or infraorbital foramen, performed most commonly on infraorbital, inferior alveolar-mental and rarely lingual nerves have been treatment used since past many years. According to latest researches, microsurgical decompression of the trigeminal root is seen to produce promising results [6].

Glossopharyngeal Neuralgia

Glossopharyngeal neuralgia is an uncommon condition, with presentation of pain, just like in trigeminal neuralgia. Pain may be triggered by talking, eating, yawning etc. with pain located in the oral and facial regions like pharynx, posterior third of tongue, soft palate, ear, border of lower jaw. In addition, patients occasionally present with bradycardia, syncope, or asystole. The incidence varies from 0.2 to 0.8 per 100,00 population per year. An equal male to female ratio with maximum incidence in 50 plus age group [7].

- Diagnosis is based on a proper history taking and a thorough clinical examination of the affected areas.
- Glossopharyngeal neuralgia can be of two types:
    1. Classic glossopharyngeal neuralgia: either idiopathic or due to vascular compression of the nerve.
    2. Secondary glossopharyngeal neuralgia: caused by trauma, tumor, surgery, or irradiation of the oropharynx.
- Apart from clinical presentation, laboratory diagnosis including tests like Erythrocyte sedimentation rate (ESR), Complete blood count (CBC), complete metabolic panel, antinuclear antibody and imaging techniques like MRI, MRA, MRN
- Treatment of glossopharyngeal neuralgia is similar to treatment of trigeminal neuralgia. Medicinal treatment (Phenytoin, carbamaze-

pine, gabapentin), nerve block with local anesthesia, with or without the addition of steroids, Rhizotomy are some of the effective ways to manage the disease.

Persistent Idiopathic Facial Pain (Atypical Odontalgia/ Phantom Facial Pain/Atypical Facial Pain)

Persistent idiopathic facial pain (PIFP) is defined as constant facial and/or oral pain with varying presentations, persisting for atleast 2 hours per day and lasting for more than 3 months [2] PIFP is a rare condition with an incidence of 4.4 per 100,000 years and prevalence of 0.03%.

Diagnosis is clinical with more than 80% of patients with a recent history of dental treatment [8].

Burning or throbbing unilateral pain which is poorly localized, deep and persistent.

Apart from Clinical presentation diagnostic aids include – Radiographs (panoramic or periapical) and MRN [9].

Management includes the use of low-dose antiseizure medications (eg, gabapentin or tricyclic antidepressants) and topical medications such as capsaicin. Laser treatment CT guided injections have been some other treatment modalities employed.

Burning Mouth Syndrome

As the name suggests, patient of burning mouth syndrome presents with an annoying burning type of pain in a clinically normal and healthy oral mucosa. The pain is usually bilateral and the most common site is the tip of tongue, but it can present on other oral mucosal surfaces.

The disease is idiopathic however factors such as stress, anxiety, depression, psychiatric disorders, hormonal dysfunction, and neuropathy, might play some role. This syndrome has a female predilection with female to male ratio of 5:1 to 7:1 and the disorder is especially seen in post-menopausal women [10].

There is no investigation diagnostic and the diagnosis is basically a diagnosis of exclusion whereby other causes of pain are excluded and the diagnosis is made if the symptoms occur for more than two hours per day for at least 3 months [2].

Management includes topical or systemic drugs like alpha lipoic acid, low-dose clonazepam, topical capsaicin; gabapentin; amitriptyline; and doxepin [11]. Other treatment strategies used are low-level laser therapy, stress, and behavioral management.

Cluster Headache

This is a type of cephalgia or pain in the head, face and neck region, with pain coming in clusters and around the same time every day for few weeks to several months, followed by pain-free periods. The pain is so annoying that patients may have develop deep anxiety, depression and even suicidal tendencies. Patients report with a severe unilateral pain of sudden onset in the temporal/periorbital area, occurring about 1 to 8 times daily or alternate days. The pain attack lasts for few minutes to few hours. There may be associated nasal congestion, runny nose, teary eyes, edema of eyelids, drooping eyelids, and bloodshot eyes. The prevalence is 0.1%, seen more common in young males with average age of 30 years, and more prominent in spring weather [12].

Risk factors include alcohol, tobacco, and nitroglycerine intake. Diagnosis is clinical with investigations like MRI or MRA to rule out brain/ pituitary mass.

Management includes preventing triggers, like tobacco and alcohol, and daily use of pharmacologic agents such as verapamil, topiramate, short-term corticosteroids, and lithium. Triptans (subcutaneous or intranasal) are effective in the treatment of acute episodes. Sublingual ergotamine and 100% hyerbaric oxygen have also been used successful to alleviate acute pain. Fremanezumab and galcanezumab are monoclonal CGRP antibodies currently being considered as investigational drugs in the treatment.

Parkinson's Disease (PD)

In 1817, James Parkinson, an English surgeon described a condition he termed "the shaking palsy," with tremor at rest, rigidity, and bradykinesia (slowness of movement), today referred to as PD. PD is a progressive neurodegenerative condition of neurons that produce dopamine, primarily located in the substantia nigra. Parkinson's usually develops in patients after the age of 50, affecting men and women equally. It is caused by a continual breakdown of neurons in the brain, decreasing the dopamine and decreasing muscular function over time [13]. These patients exhibit tremors as well as muscular stiffness. Some of the oral manifestations include: drooling, muscle aches, muscular atrophy, and difficulty swallowing. The tremors and inability to keep their mouths open may cause a challenge to receiving dental care. Some Parkinson's medications will affect saliva as well as blood pressure. Special care will be required in managing these patients. Presence of tremor alleviates against effective oral hygiene and plaque control measures. Weakened swallowing capability can augment the risk of aspiration (choking) of sophisticated dental instruments. In addition, people with Parkinson's disease who have been on prescriptions like levodopa for several years may begin to develop dyskinesias, which can affect the jaw (where they are called orobuccal dyskinesias) as well as teeth grinding [14]. Individuals suffering from Parkinson's disease may also experience dry mouth or xerostomia, with consequences on the oral status and oral mucosa that frequently lead to the worsening of already existing masticatory difficulties or denture anxiety. As the normal salivary flow helps to maintain the integrity of the oral mucosa, reduction of the salivary flow severely compromises the remineralization process of oral hard tissues and new dental caries possibly will easily appear including root surface caries [15]. Dry mouth condition also lowers the resistance of the oral mucous membrane to the foreign body invasion. This is especially true for trauma caused by the loosening of dentures due to the lack of the saliva as salivary biofilm is desirable for the perfect adhesion.

Multiple Sclerosis (MS)

MS, the most common autoimmune disease of the central nervous system (CNS), is a complex neurological condition. It is a disease of muscular control, affecting more women than men, usually diagnosed between the ages of 20 and 40. It is a degenerative disease, caused by inflammatory damage to the nerve sheath, exhibiting muscle weakness over time. Dental/Maxillofacial patients may exhibit delayed motor skills, drooling, ptosis, tremors, lack of balance, and lack of motor control [16]. Some facial paralysis may develop and affect the ability to perform proper oral hygiene procedures and may affect the ability to retain removable prostheses.

Cerebral Palsy

Cerebral palsy affects both the brain and the nervous system, and it may be manifested any time from early infancy. It is due to an injury or abnormality in the brain. This usually does not get worse over time. Different types of cerebral palsy exist and patients may exhibit a variety of symptoms. Patients may exhibit tremors, muscular and joint tightening, an unsteady gait, and weak musculature. Patients with cerebral palsy may exhibit more malocclusion, bruxism, and hypocalcification, as well as oral injuries caused by falling due to concomitant muscular issues [17]. Some of these patients may be on antiseizure medication, which has the potential to affect gingival growth.

Muscular Dystrophy

Muscular dystrophy is a genetic condition that exhibits loss of muscle tissue, leading to muscular weakness, which worsens over time. Affected muscles may be localized (pelvis, shoulder, or face) or may be more widespread throughout the body. There are several types of muscular dystrophy. Myotonic will affect chewing and the ability to move lips and turn one's head. Patients may experience malocclusion and TMD due to the muscular weakness [18].

Huntington's Disease

Huntington's disease may exhibit uncontrollable movements due to nerve cells in certain parts of the brain degrading and degenerating. It is a genetic defect of chromosome four, which causes a section of DNA to repeat several times [19]. Patients tend to develop symptoms between the ages of 30 and 40, but, rarely, it may occur in younger children or adolescents. Patients may exhibit unusual movements including grimacing, head turning, abnormal gait, and wild movements of the extremities. They also lack muscular control of the face and tongue. Swallowing is also an issue. Oral hygiene may be quite difficult due to the uncontrollable movements.

Myasthenia Gravis

Myasthenia gravis is an autoimmune neuromuscular disorder. The etiology is unknown but it may be due to a tumor of the thymus. It can occur at any age though it is more common in young women and older men. Patients experience partial or no facial expressions because of facial paralysis. These patients have muscle weakness in their tongues as well as palates, making swallowing and chewing difficult. Patients may also experience breathing difficulties due to weakened muscles of the chest wall, as well as a droopy head.

Dysphagia

Swallowing, as we know, is a multisystem event. It involves proper musculature and nerve transmission to the brain, as well as assistance by the teeth in mastication and the salivary glands in lubrication and enzymatic action on food. Furthermore, it will be affected by any issues affecting the larynx or esophagus. Dysphagia, or difficulty swallowing, usually affects older adults although it can also affect babies. Forty percent of nursing home residents are affected by this malady. Dysphagia has many etiologies. Dysphagia may be caused by an actual blockage, such as GERD (gastroesophageal reflux disease) or the inability of the muscles to conduct peristalsis due to an underlying neurological disease such as muscular dystrophy, Parkinson's, or multiple sclerosis [20]. Patients with dysphagia will exhibit symptoms of difficulty swallowing, may have issues with chewing due to lack of swallowing function, or have problems moving food from their mouth and through their esophagus. They may feel as if they have a lump in their throat. They may also exhibit malnutrition, dehydration, as well as aspiration of food particles due to coughing and choking as they try to clear their esophagus.

These patients need to be seen by their physician to determine the etiology of their swallowing dysfunction. We may see them before they realize they have a swallowing issue. We may notice food and material buildup on the tooth surfaces as well as noncleared food from the oral cavity. Patients may exhibit frequent dry coughing or attempts to clear their throat at times not surrounding meals.

Hypoglossal Nerve Injury

The twelfth cranial nerve, which controls tongue movement, is the hypoglossal nerve. Hypoglossal nerve injury is also usually unilateral, with the tongue deviating to the affected side. Unilateral atrophy of the tongue may be a sign after prolonged injury to this nerve. Etiology of hypoglossal nerve injury may also be caused by tumors, stroke, or any of the degenerative diseases affecting muscles and nerves. Patients will have difficulty speaking, talking, and chewing with both of these conditions. Oral hygiene may be affected as well as oral clearance.

Bell's Palsy

Bell's palsy as well as hypoglossal nerve injury may be caused by a dental injection or a tumor. Both will have an effect on the patient's condition. Both may be temporary or longer lasting, depending on the etiology. With Bell's palsy, which affects the seventh cranial (or facial) nerve, only one side of the patient's face is affected. There may be a rapid onset of mild weakness to a full-blown facial paralysis. Facial expression may be affected by the weakness of the muscles, in addition to a sensation of pain or increased sensitivity on the affected side. Headaches are not uncommon. Taste may be affected. Lyme disease or herpetic lesions may also cause Bell's palsy.

Conclusion

These disorders are by no means a complete list. There are always untoward reactions to medications or disease states that may cause issues with the oral cavity. Xerostomia due to medications or aging may cause symptoms that mimic neuromuscular diseases. Some senior patients may exhibit symptoms of xerostomia, slight tremors, and lack of dexterity or slowness in gait without a concomitant neurological or muscular-based disorder.

References

[1] Iwata K., Sessle B. J. The Evolution of Neuroscience as a Research Field Relevant to Dentistry. *Journal of Dental Research.* 2019;98(13):1407-1417. doi: https://10.1177/0022034519875724.

[2] Headache Classification Committee of the International Headache Society (IHS). The International Classification of Headache Disorders, 3rd edition (beta version). *Cephalalgia.* 2013 Jul;33(9):629-808. doi: https://10.1177/0 33 3102413485658. PMID: 23771276.

[3] Shankar Kikkeri N., Nagalli S. Trigeminal Neuralgia. [Updated 2021 Jul 5]. In: *StatPearls* [Internet]. Treasure Island (FL): StatPearls Publishing; 2021 Jan-. Available from: https://www.ncbi.nlm.nih.gov/books/NBK554486/.

[4] Sanders R. D. The Trigeminal (V) and Facial (VII) Cranial Nerves: Head and Face Sensation and Movement. *Psychiatry (*Edgmont). 2010 Jan;7(1): 13-6. PMID: 20386632; PMCID: PMC2848459.

[5] Maarbjerg S., Di Stefano G., Bendtsen L., Cruccu G. Trigeminal Neuralgia - Diagnosis and Treatment. *Cephalalgia.* 2017;37(7):648-657. doi: https://10.1177/0333102416687280.

[6] Al-Quliti K. W. Update on Neuropathic Pain Treatment for Trigeminal Neuralgia. The Pharmacological and Surgical Options. *Neurosciences* (Riyadh). 2015 Apr;20(2):107-14. doi: https://10.17712/nsj.2015.2.20 14 0501.PMID: 25864062; PMCID: PMC4727618.

[7] Shah R. J., Padalia D. Glossopharyngeal Neuralgia. [Updated 2021 Feb 24]. In: *StatPearls* [Internet]. Treasure Island (FL): StatPearls Publishing; 2021 Jan-. Available from: https://www.ncbi.nlm.nih.gov/books/NBK541041/.

[8] Ziegeler, C., Schulte, Laura H. A. B., May, Arnea, Altered Trigeminal Pain Processing on Brainstem Level in Persistent Idiopathic Facial Pain, *Pain*: May 2021 - Volume 162 - Issue 5 - p 1374-1378 doi: https://10.1097/j.pain.0000000000002126.

[9] Park H. O., Ha J. H., Jin M. U., Kim Y. K., Kim S. K. Diagnostic Challenges of Nonodontogenic Toothache. *Restor Dent Endod.* 2012;37(3):170-174. doi:https://10.5395/rde.2012.37.3.170.

[10] Dahiya P., Kamal R., Kumar M., Niti, Gupta R., Chaudhary K. Burning Mouth Syndrome and Menopause. *Int J Prev Med.* 2013;4(1):15-20.

[11] Feller L., Fourie J., Bouckaert M., Khammissa R. A. G., Ballyram R., Lemmer J. Burning Mouth Syndrome: Aetiopathogenesis and Principles of Management. *Pain Res Manag.* 2017;2017:1926269. doi: https://10.1155/2 017/1926269.

[12] Wei D. Y., Yuan Ong J. J., Goadsby P. J. Cluster Headache: Epidemiology, Pathophysiology, Clinical Features, and Diagnosis. *Ann Indian Acad Neurol.* 2018;21(Suppl 1):S3-S8. doi: https://10.4103/aian.AIAN_349_17.

[13] Cerri S., Mus L., Blandini F. Parkinson's Disease in Women and Men: What's the Difference? *J Parkinsons Dis.* 2019;9(3):501-515. doi: https://1 0.3233/JPD-191683.

[14] Raoofi S., Khorshidi H., Najafi M. Etiology, Diagnosis and Management of Oromandibular Dystonia: An Update for Stomatologists. *J Dent* (Shiraz). 2017;18(2):73-81.

[15] Abou Neel E. A., Aljabo A., Strange A., et al., Demineralization-Remineralization Dynamics in Teeth and Bone. *Int J Nanomedicine*. 2016;11:4743-4763. Published 2016 Sep 19. doi: https://10.2147/IJN.S 107624.

[16] Doty R. L., MacGillivray M. R., Talab H., Tourbier I., Reish M., Davis S., Cuzzocreo J. L., Shepard N. T., Pham D. L. Balance in Multiple Sclerosis: Relationship to Central Brain Regions. *Exp Brain Res.* 2018 Oct;236(10):2739-2750. doi: https://10.1007/s00221-018-5332-1. Epub 2018 Jul 17. PMID: 30019234.

[17] Jan B. M., Jan M. M. Dental Health of Children with Cerebral Palsy. *Neurosciences* (Riyadh). 2016;21(4):314-318. doi: https://10.17712/nsj.20 16.4.20150729.

[18] McDonald C. M. Clinical Approach to the Diagnostic Evaluation of Hereditary and Acquired Neuromuscular Diseases. *Phys Med Rehabil Clin N Am.* 2012;23(3):495-563. doi: https://10.1016/j.pmr.2012.06.011.

[19] Paulson H. L., Albin R. L. Huntington's Disease: Clinical Features and Routes to Therapy. In: *Neurobiology of Huntington's Disease: Applications to Drug Discovery*. [Internet]. Boca Raton (FL): CRC Press/Taylor & Francis; 2011. Chapter 1. Available from: https://www.ncbi.nlm.ni h.gov/b ooks/NBK56000/.

[20] Sura L., Madhavan A., Carnaby G., Crary M. A. Dysphagia in the elderly: management and nutritional considerations. *Clin Interv Aging*. 2012;7:287-298. doi: https://10.2147/CIA.S23404.

Chapter 12

Neurolaw: The Legal Perspective of Neuroscience

Yashi Garg* **and Rachit Gupta**
Yashi Garg and Associates, Lucknow, India

Abstract

The validity of the claims is the foundation of scientific theory evolution through a thorough methodology that covers all areas of neuroscience. Law is no exception to this scientific principle too. The intersection of law and neuroscience, with the brain as a common correlative element, gives rise to neurolaw as an interdisciplinary field that provides a more thorough and accurate understanding of legal issues. The research of neurolaw can be studied under three basis areas – Intervention, Assessment, and Revision. Civil and Criminal responsibility litigation, problems of establishing neuroscientific findings as evidence which are among the practical concerns in the courtroom or neuro-litigation issues, are the focus of neurolaw practical researchers. In the theoretical approach, we comprehend the brain and its functioning in terms of conceptual worth. Such an approach is especially important for highlighting the influence of the brain on behavior. The Judicial System of India has taken notice of this rapidly developing science in the criminal justice system. Since the early twentieth century, the use of neuroscience has been in legal procedures. The most important question in this field of neuroscience is how it is and will be employed in the legal system, just as, neurolaw attempts to relate neuro-ethics to moral principles as well as it relates the brain to the law. Neurolaw provides opportunities for psychiatry. Therefore, "One of the most likely methods for neuroscience

* Corresponding Author's Email: yashigarg0491@gmail.com.

In: New Perspectives in Neuroscience
Editors: Prachi Srivastava, Neha Srivastava and Prekshi Garg
ISBN: 978-1-68507-754-9

to help the legal system" is the insanity defense. Hence, the goal of neurolaw research is to strike a compromise between two issues – Overenthusiasm and Over-criticism. If there is active participation by the psychiatrists in the field of development, the chances of success will improve.

Introduction

The validity of the claims is the foundation of scientific theory evolution through a thorough methodology that covers all areas of neuroscience [1]. Law is no exception to this scientific principle too.

Usually, legal effects and repercussions are linked to neurological concerns, thus a call to neuroscience for a clearer explanation of legal principles is unavoidable. The intersection of law and neuroscience, with the brain as a common correlative element, gives rise to neurolaw as an interdisciplinary field that provides a more thorough and accurate understanding of legal issues. All of this contributes to more accurate legal evidence and a more equitable justice system. Additionally, neurolaw contributes to the expansion of both sciences.

There are numerous instances where neuroscientific data could be useful in better understanding legal concerns. This is why, in practice, a growing number of neuroscientific pieces of evidence are reaching courts in a variety of legal circumstances. Neurolaw would give rise to a more intelligent and effective judiciary, legislative, and executive system. Neuroscience breakthroughs have the potential to change legal provisions, as well as procedural legislation and conventions, or perhaps completely transform them into something new.

The Intersection of Neuroscience and Law: Neurolaw

Scientists who have led research on the human brain extensively have known a great deal about how it functions, how it malfunctions, and how it may be fixed or transformed. Neuroscience, or the study of the nervous system from a scientific standpoint, is a comparatively new field that has already changed medical practices. Neuroscience is nowadays an interdisciplinary science that works with other results [2]. It was also an instant and significant motivator for understanding how the neurological system operates and how it affects neurolaw [3].Neurolaw is an effort to understand the link between law and the brain by using insights from neuroscience [4]. Neurolaw investigates the ramifications of neuroscience discoveries on legal laws [5].

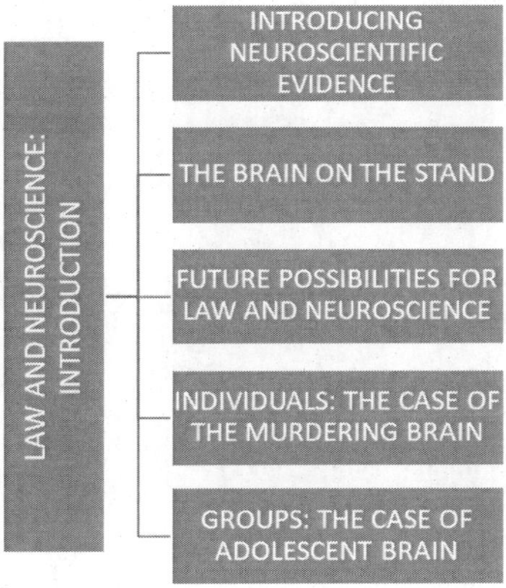

Figure 1. Law and neurosciences.

The possibility of a link between law and neuroscience is the most fundamental question among neuroscientists and lawyers. Law is a humanities science based on obligations, arising from collective wisdom and abstract propositions, whereas neuroscience is a natural science based on experiments and indicative statements. As many legal academics agree, the law is a social phenomenon shaped by the social compact. As a result, the law is based on relative concepts, whereas neuroscience is based on absolute notions. This raises the question of how it is possible to create and defend "Neurolaw". The law is human's innovative way [6] of regulating individuals' conduct in an insecure and unstable community, rather than in a natural community where there is no law, no state, people do whatever they want, and security is minimized [7]. The ultimate goal of the law is to protect human dignity to realize a person's humanity and achieve true justice. This objective can be achieved if society's laws are better and more accurate. To put it in another way, we need a more equitable justice system. Neuroscientific assertions, in addition to an acute understanding of neurological phenomena, aid law in developing more precise laws in this area. Neurolaw, moreover, throws light on the justice path for law in its scientific field. For example, when legislators want to pass a specific law to penalize offenders, or when courts want to decide on an accused person, neurological advances provide lawyers with precise glasses that allow them to get a sense of the overall picture and make it more equitable and fair legal decisions.

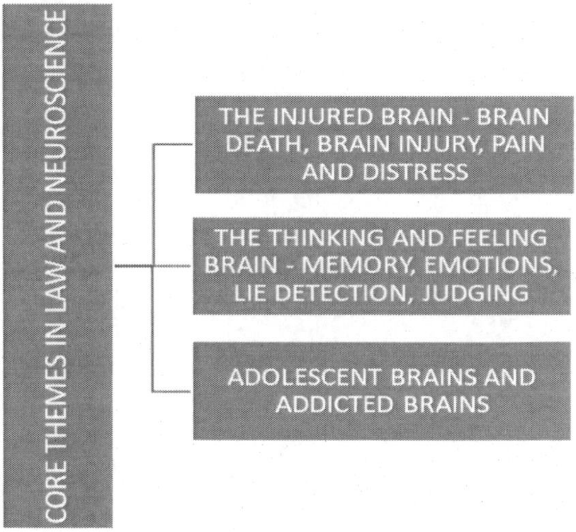

Figure 2. The core themes in law and neuroscience.

Neurolawyers use neuroscience to try to understand human behavior, and they may help to define future legal processes. In practice, they deliberate on medical technology scanning of the human brain and nervous systems, like radiology, psychiatry, neurology, and clinical neuropsychology [8]. Researchers interested in the human brain's operation now have an unprecedented chance to investigate the neurobiological aspects of human behavior, thanks to these novel imaging techniques. In essence, neuroimaging approaches provide visual brain demarcation, which is then interpreted by an imaging specialist. [9] In the beginning, the field of neuroscience has been used in procedural law to support criminal and civil responsibility claims in court.

Despite this practical use, the field of neuroscience has been used in a variety of legal subfields. Today, neuroscientific concepts are being incorporated into a variety of legal fields, including Intellectual Property Law, Tort Law, Consumer Law, Health Law, Employment Law, Constitutional Law, and Criminal Law [10]. Even other allied sciences, like psychology, sociology, political science, behavioral ecology, and economics, pervade the purview of neurolaw, which focuses mostly on criminology [11].

The Intersection of Neurosciences and Criminal Laws

Outside of the legal setting, there are various more neurolaw discoveries that interested readers should be aware of. The MacArthur Foundation, for example, has contributed more than $ 15 million in the Law and Neuroscience Project (2007-2011, based at the University of California, Santa Barbara) and the Research Network on Law and Neuroscience (2011-2014 based at Vanderbilt University).

The organization's main goal has been to form collaborations between neuroscientists, judges, and legal scholars to:

- Direct the legal system in identifying the promise of neuroscientific understandings while avoiding the pitfalls of interpreting them.
- Conduct new, collaborative, interdisciplinary research that can assist in the improvement of the Criminal Justice System's fairness and effectiveness.

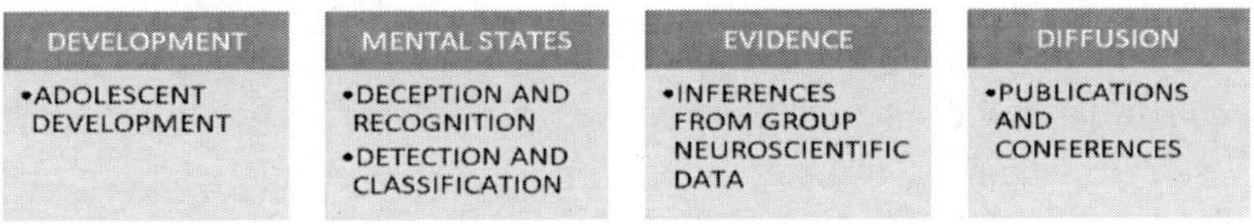

Figure 3. The intersection of neurosciences and criminal law.

Neuroscience has provided light on how the brain and certain mental processes work, and it is created on a comprehension of the brain's structure and function. Because the law is primarily concerned with regulating people's behavior, it provides insight into the mental processes that underline human behavior. It shapes neurolaw, an interdisciplinary discipline. There is no direct mapping of mental function in certain areas of the brain [12] because of substantial variances in people's brains [13]. In the field of neurolaw, this is a major challenge. Neurolaw scientists are attempting to apply neurological findings to legal rules and systems for the purpose to improve legal standards, norms, and practices. More specifically, the unique neuroscientific approach to legality of rules and consequences results in an even perfect and better representation of legal effects, as a result, the laws governing them are mutated, allowing for a more thorough legal system to be obeyed.

Neurolaw Research Domains

There are three basic areas of research in neurolaw that can be identified:

- Revision
- Assessment
- Intervention [14]

Revision

In the revision arena, researchers are investigating whether neurological results should lead to changes in the law and legal processes. The idea that neuroscience studies reveal free will is an illusion and that no one should be held legally accountable since free will is regarded to be crucial for accountability is well-known, if not renowned, for example. This debate is being made as an origin for a substantial change of criminal law that eliminates the fundamentals of vengeance and guilt. Since no offender is ever criminally culpable, this kind of change can also suggest that the irrationality defense is no longer relevant. As a result, at least in terms of the elements of criminal responsibility, defendants' mental evaluations would become obsolete.

Assessment

The appraisal of persons is the second research domain. Individuals in criminal law, such as defendants, inmates, witnesses, and potential jurors, are frequently interested in their mental states.

For example, lawyers may be asked to respond to the following questions:

- Is the defendant afflicted with a mental illness?
- Is he legally mad or incompetent to face his charges?
- What is the likelihood of this particular prisoner recidivism?
- Is the witness lying about what he/she remembers?
- Is the potential juror prejudiced towards specific groups?

These problems may be solved in the future using neuroscience approaches – to say the least, this is the key area of neurolaw research. The accuracy with which a lie is detected has long been a source of contention, and a brain-based counterpart is most likely to be no different – yet, regardless of the dispute, the company "No Lie MRI" is already up and running [15].

One of the most important legal questions with mind-reading procedures is whether they can be employed against a person's will and if yes, then, under what circumstances [16].

Intervention

The third research area is concerned with neuroscientific therapies. In this regard, there is currently very little that can be done. However, it is hoped and frequently expected, for example, that neuroscience will lead to therapeutic alternatives which minimize the probability of repetition. An article on deep brain stimulation (DBS) to diminish sexual drive, that could be used in sexual offenders, was recently published in this journal [17]. Such brain-based therapies may become available in the future, raising a dozen of new problems. There are other potentials for intervention as well, such as criminals gaining access to brain equipment. Someday, anti-heroes may try to use neuro-techniques to persuade others into doing crimes. They could gain access to a person's DBS device, which is used to treat obsessive-compulsive disorder [18]. Can an individual whose brain has been tampered with to commit a crime be held legally liable, and if yes, then, under what circumstances?

There are only a few of the fascinating questions that could be found in the three areas of neurolaw research. Neurolaw researchers, thus, do not have to be neuro-enthusiasts. Instead, they could be quite hostile to the use of neuroscience in the courtroom.

A Reflection on Two Main Types of Research in Neurolaw

While the brain decade [19] was first brought to the medical and legal professions, neurolaw is a relatively recent and highly interdisciplinary field. Taylor et al. were the first to coin the term "neurolaw' among legal scholars [20]. He raised the problem more effectively with his well-known scholarly scientific paper called "Neuropsychologists and Neurolawyers". Taylor's contributions in the field of neurolaw, particularly legal practices, during his academic career [21] are of considerable significance. Neuroscience and law have a lengthy history of interaction. However, since 1990, neuroscientists and neurolawyers have frequently disagreed regarding the likelihood of neurolaw spreading. This topic is also regularly discussed by lecturers at scientific conferences in the United States, the United Kingdom, France, and Canada [22].

Practical Researches

Civil and Criminal responsibility litigation, problems of establishing neuroscientific findings as evidence which are among the practical concerns in the courtroom or neuro-litigation issues, are the focus of neurolaw practical researchers.

In the field of neurolaw, there is a lot of legal procedural literature. One of the most recent noteworthy publications is "Neuroscience and Legal Responsibility" [23]. It takes a broadly compatibilist approach for the study of legal responsibility. How could neuroscience, psychology, and behavioral genetics influence legal responsibility procedures, according to the author? In this study, established notions of free choice and legal culpability are primarily challenged.

"International Neurolaw: A Comparative Analysis" [24], along with some other works, compares the dissimilar lawful arrangements and policies that they suggest for dealing with neurolaw implications, as a result, it is critical to understand different legal approaches to revise lawful systems in light of new neuroscience findings.

Moreover, these are some more useful works that might help solve problems in legal practice:

1. "Neurolaw for Trial Lawyers," [25]
2. "Law and Neuroscience: Current Legal Issues," [26]
3. "Neuroscience in the Courtroom," [27]
4. "A Primer on Criminal Law and Neuroscience." [28]

These publications have a strong emphasis on practical lawful regulation and technical law, both of which are influenced by neurolaw. Practical neurolaw is most closely tied to neuro-litigation, which involves judges and lawyers using one of the latest criminal procedural law rules in the courtroom.

According to what was addressed, these are the important subjects that have been planned in neurolaw practical research:

- Neuro-litigation trials,
- Tools based on neuroscience that can be used to prove or disprove legal culpability,
- Neuro-criminology in Procedural law,
- Standing neuro-litigation,
- Neuro advocacy and attorney,
- Neuroscience and judgment,
- Right to appeal for brain injury.

Theoretical Researches

In the theoretical approach, on the other hand, we comprehend the brain and its functioning in terms of conceptual worth. Such an approach is especially important for highlighting the influence of the brain on behavior. By doing so, we are recognizing new laws in the judicial system that regulate these behaviors. The use of neuroscience discoveries in judicial procedures has expanded as neuroscientific tools contribute to a better comprehension of the mind. Cognitive neuroscientists study the interplay between the mind and the brain. They do it instead by employing cutting-edge techniques like fMRI and electroencephalography (EEG). As a result, neuroscientific research and technology are being used to improve judicial system norms and processes based on inferences taken from these discoveries and increasingly advanced technologies. In this regard, contemporary philosophical concerns raise conceptual underpinnings of neurolaw. Theoretical researchers investigate the reasons in favor of the greater use of neuroscience in the legal system. They deplete the resources available for determining its creditability in judicial processes. In addition, theorists strive to incorporate neuroscientific knowledge into substantive legal concepts. As a result, these impacts encompass a wide range of theoretical and practical challenges.

The books listed below are maybe the most notable ones based on this research strategy.

1. "Minds, Brains, and Law: The Conceptual Foundations of Law and Neuroscience," [29]

2. "Neurolaw: Brain and Spinal Cord Injuries," [30]
3. "Law, Mind and Brain," [31]
4. "Materials on Neurolaw," [32]
5. "Law and the Brain" [33]
6. "The Neurobiology of Criminal Behaviour." [34]

Thus, mentioned below are the important studies in the subject of neurolaw theoretical research:

- Possibility of incorporating neuroscience findings into the legal system,
- The brain and the law are two concepts that are often used interchangeably,
- The link between the brain and the law,
- In the legal system and the future, neuroscience technologies, and development,
- Disordered legal orders and brain illness,
- On the legal liability of mental illness and brain injury,
- The right to privacy and the use of brain imaging,
- Third-party punishment is a matter of personal choice,
- Neuroscience and legal rights,
- Neuroscience and legal freedoms,
- Brain injury citizenship rights,
- Individuals' right to security about people with neurological diseases,
- Impact of neurolaw theories on legal regulations.

Contribution of Neurolaw to Judiciary

The Judicial System of India has taken notice of this rapidly developing science in the criminal justice system [35]. The case state of Maharashtra v Sharma [36] demonstrates that the Indian Judicial System has been aggressive in incorporating neuroscience into the legal system. This was a murder case, and the woman was convicted based on circumstantial evidence [37] such as a brain mapping/scan [38]. This was a contentious decision that drew criticism from the judicial community. Prof Hank Greely of Sandford University criticized the state of Maharashtra v Sharma judgment, stating that the BEOSP [39] process is not universally approved by the scientists around the world, and the end products are not 100% accurate, so there should be evident proof to back up viewpoints/findings based on BEOSP. The critical study could be good for such studies since more criticism will be beneficial to identify the flaws and knowing all of this would aid scientists in developing a perfect brain mapping machine [40].

Though neuroscience evidence is not commonly utilized in criminal cases, it is on the rise, as seen in this graph of US Judicial opinions referencing a defendant's use of neuroscience.

There are some defenses, such as insanity and brain death, where the scanning of a brain will not give the desired results, however, in the instance of a false insanity defense, the scanning of the brain can be an important tool to determine the culprit's liability. The accompanying image depicts the behavior of a killer and a healthy participant, as well as scanning of the brain that shows vivid red and yellow colors indicating activation of high brain and black and blue colors indicating low activation. The illustration above aids judicial officials in determining responsibility.

Functional Magnet Resonance Imaging [41] (FMRI) monitors the activity of the human brain and creates pictures of living areas in the brain that are involved with the usage of machines where a person thinks, reacts, or accomplishes anything with the support of the computer software.

Brain Electrical Oscillation Signature Profiling (BEOSP) Evidentiary Value

In the year 2003, the Brain Electrical Oscillation Signature Profiling methodology was created. Three cities in India provide BEOSP techniques – Mumbai, Chandigarh, and Gandhinagar. More than 300 people were put through a brain electrical oscillation signature profiling examination to see if their statements as defendants in various crimes remained credible.

Section 45 of the Indian Evidence Act of 1872 [42] was used to summon suspects. Specific methodologies were studied and acted as a foundation for evaluations, which were made using a BEOS system and the results were examined qualitatively. FMRI and BEOS are two novel neuroscientific approaches that are directing the court in the investigation process. These procedures have been applied on over 300 subjects, but on no single occasion have they been the primary factor in making a choice.

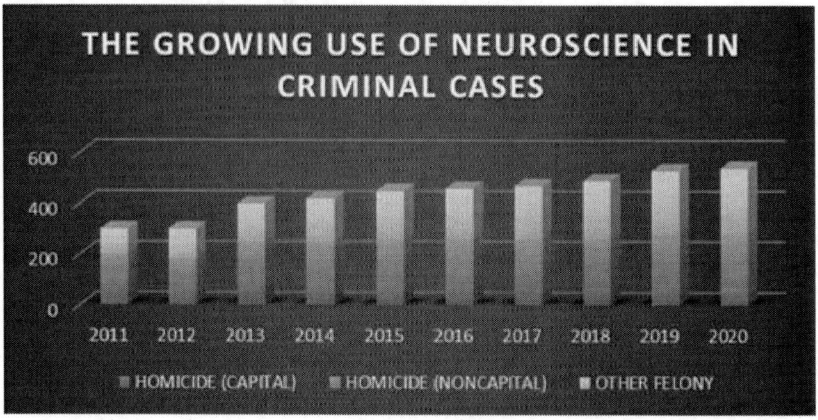

Figure 4. The trend of the growing use of neuroscience in criminal cases.

According to section 45of the Indian Evidence Act 1872, expert advice on various subjects, particularly science and art, is permissible. Thus, it opens the door to the use of neuroscientific methods in the examination procedure. Technically, conclusions based on BEOS or other neuroscience techniques are beneficial because it aids the investigation agency in obtaining information and other evidence that will be useful to the court in deciding a case.

BEOS is not a panacea for all the issues, courts employ it only in specific cases where material evidence is lacking and there is no other way to obtain it, such as cases involving terrorism, mafia, high-profile scams as well as other instances where the accused is afraid to speak the truth. As a result, BEOS approaches [43] would be extremely useful in these situations.

Applicability of Neuroscience in Courtroom

Since the early twentieth century, the use of neuroscience has been in legal procedures. Shen dates one of the earliest applications of neuroscience in the courtroom to the 1940s when EEG was initially employed in a case involving an epileptic defendant. When EEG was utilized to throw some light on the subject of identifying and treating epilepsy, few lawyers used it to argue against laws that denied epilepsy patients' rights, whereas some others used it to try to uncover the violence-related brain markers. EEG had become so common in the cases related to epilepsy by the mid-twentieth century that psychiatrist and attorney Irwin Perr advised, "The lawyer interested in this subject must know some principles of electroencephalography, both in understanding and evaluating epilepsy and because it is frequently used as a mechanism in court cases." Indeed, attorneys were advised to learn EEG within a few decades of its invention, both for its probative significance and its expanding prominence in the courtroom.

President Ronald Reagan's attempted assassination by John Hinckley in 1981 resulted in one of the most high-profile cases involving the request of neuroscience in unlawful prosecution. Hinckley's defense squad used a Computed Tomography (CT) scan of his brain to back up their assertion that the person had schizophrenia and hence should not be judged guilty because of insanity (NGRI). Despite the prosecution's objections to Hinckley's CT scan being admitted as evidence, the district court judge ordered that they were permissible. Hinckley was eventually discovered NGRI.

A decade later, in People v Weinstein, a new kind of neuroimaging was introduced. Weinstein was charged with second-degree murder, after strangling his wife and hurling her from their Manhattan Apartment's 12th floor, a crime he willingly acknowledged to. His lawyers considered it mistrustful that Weinstein would express such slight sorrow for his deeds, so they well-ordered PET scans. At experimental, Weinstein's defense team presented his PET scans to support their allegation that his brain function was affected due to an arachnoid cyst. As a result, they asserted that the accused lacked the mental capacity to be deemed criminally accountable. Weinstein was ultimately permitted to plead embarrassed to the reduced custody of assassination.

Neuroscience-based criminal defenses are most common in first-degree murder trials, but they are not confined to these crimes [44].

The regulations limiting the admission of scientific evidence into the federal prosecutions altered dramatically only a year after the Weinstein case. Two families sued Merrell Dow Pharmaceuticals, Inc. in Daubert v. Merrell Dow Pharmaceuticals, Inc. for their kids' birth abnormalities, which were purportedly instigated by prenatal intake of a drug traded by the firm. Even though the district court awarded summary judgment for Merrell Dow, the families filed an appeal, and the case was eventually considered by the United States Supreme Court. Before Daubert, judges who preside over trials utilized the "Frye Standard" to determine whether scientific testimony was admissible. The Frye standard required that the procedure for gathering evidence was gathered be "generally accepted" by the applicable technical community for testimony to be accepted for trial. Congress had created the Federal Rules of Evidence (FRE) about two decades before Daubert, which set a softer approach bar for permitting scientific testimony to be used in court. Rather than needing "general acceptance" of the scientific process for acceptability, the FRE's criterion considered it to be simply one of several factors to evaluate, including whether the approach is testable, whether it has been peer-reviewed, and its known or prospective error rate. The Supreme Court overturned Frye's primacy in federal proceedings in Daubert, replacing it with the FRE's test, which has become known as the "Daubert standard." This allowed for a more-free application of scientific evidence in modern courts. The Daubert standard, in particular, allowed scientific methodologies and results that had not yet gained widespread recognition to be used in courtrooms. As a result, new imaging methods that were not extensively utilized before, become acceptable [45].

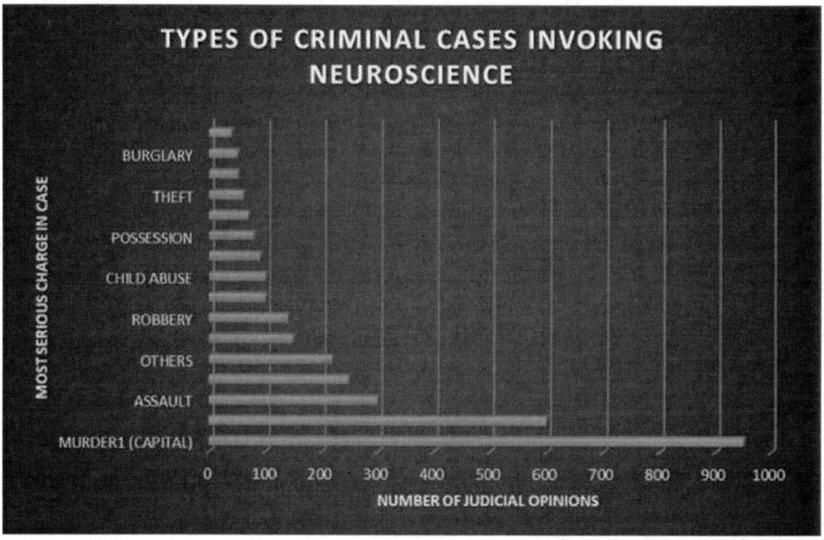

Figure 5. Type of criminal cases invoking neuroscience

Some of the Encountering Questions That Are Faced by the Neurolawyers

The most important question in this field of neuroscience is how it is and will be employed in the legal system, just as, neurolaw attempts to relate neuro-ethics to moral principles as well as it relates the brain to the law. A wide variety of possible neuroscience and legal intersections are presented by scientists [46]. As it emerges, neuroscience can benefit law in a variety of ways (including at the very least in the contexts of Buttressing, Challenging, Detecting, Sorting, Intervening, Explaining, and Predicting) [47]. In a practical sense, evidence indicates the large number of situations that have neuroscientific ramifications which are increasing rapidly. As a result, this necessitates a broad understanding of both law and neuroscience. As a result, many problems remained unsolved, such as:

- To what extent is it possible that the brain may influence human behavior in a certain way that has legal implications?
- What legal standards and precedents should cover this part of a set of rules to create a fairer and more equal legal system?
- What role can neuroscience have in civil and criminal law?

Moreover, neurolaw addresses moral issues concerning nootropics, sometimes called mind-altering medications. Neural, Memory, Intelligence Enhancers (functional foods, supplements, and nutraceuticals that boost one or more areas of mental processing, like working memory, motivation, and focus) [48] and Cognitive are referred to as nootropics, that is smart drugs. Thus, many problems remained unsolved, such as:

- What impact will these enhancements have on people's legal rights in society?
- Is it necessary to use a performance-enhancing drug just simply to keep up with the rest of society?
- Do people have the right to experiment under the law with chemicals to alter their perception?

The emergence of modern neuroscience expands dramatically as a result of new technology that the law has had to deal with. It is important to be satisfied that we have sufficient knowledge to form conclusions that are legally relevant on an appropriate level. Hence, because of it, many problems remained unsolved, such as:

- Is there anything in neuroscience that we don't have any clue about from common sense or past behavioral research?
- Is it possible for scientific researchers and medical practitioners to communicate their findings in manners that are understandable to a legal audience?

- Is there any area of law where neuroscience will never make sense?
- Are we infringing on the right to privacy when we try to gain access to brain data using medical science technologies such as FMRI?
- What kind of legal norms could be set for these issues?

Thus, these difficulties are amplified much more in a theoretical sense by the statistic that legal theory and legal doctrine drawn on our everyday thinking of mental life and mind notions. Furthermore, addressing the link between Mind, Brain and Law is extremely challenging. Neurolaw theorists emphasize this by focusing on the extent and outlines of involvement of claims in neuroscience and law, using conceptual technique and a philosophical viewpoint. Also, they rely less on practical, ethical, and empirical methods. [49] The essential question in a conceptual, methodological approach is the what of the brain, mind, and law, and thus comprehending them in the genuine sense brings us to a mature abstract retrospect of behavior and manners. As a result, the way is made for a system of legal laws to govern behaviors in society.

Other Law and Neuroscience Issues Beyond Criminal Responsibility

The majority of the scholarly debate on law and neuroscience has focussed on issues of responsibility. If neuroscience can help us connect physical brain states to subjective mental states, it will be extremely beneficial. Neuroscience, on the other hand, appears to have a lot more to offer law. For example, neuroscience may assist us in learning about relevant current mental states, to boost our ability to forecast future mental states and consequent behavior, it may allow us to intervene in the brain more directly to cure non-disease behaviors, and it may lead to the discovery of new techniques to increase human mental capabilities. All of these developments will be influenced by the law, both directly and indirectly [50].

Neuroscience may improve our forecast of a person's future by making available to us a greater understanding of the physical underpinnings of diseases of neurological nature, mental diseases, and nonpathological behaviors. In certain circumstances, this is more accurately described as an early diagnosis of a disease process that has yet to manifest clear symptoms. Early detection of Alzheimer's disease symptoms, for example, using PET scans for amyloid plaque build-up or biomarkers in the cerebral spinal fluid. In other circumstances, like the link between particular genetic variations and prospective Alzheimer's disease, it could be more of a hunch. In any such case, a finer understanding of illnesses like Alzheimer's disease, Schizophrenia, Parkinson's disease, and others could help us anticipate who will be diagnosed with the illness and who will not. This has apparent legal consequences, as it will raise legal difficulties surrounding employment, insurance, education, and other benefits that may be rejected or supplied based on such forecasts. (For example, it's also possible that potential judicial appointees would be asked for medical evidence of their risk for Alzheimer's disease.) Because this understanding improves early diagnosis, it may have a more direct impact on judicial procedures, impacting decisions regarding a person's capacity to be a witness or to manage his finances, as well as other key life issues.

Neuroscience-based predictions may also have a direct impact on the legal system, as they improve our ability to forecast someone's future aggressive or criminal behavior. Predictions are already utilized in court proceedings to make decisions on bail, sentencing, parole, the death sentence, and even preventative custody in specific mental and sexual offender cases. Predictions might be subjective at times. They can also be clinical. In other cases, social science evidence has been used to construct predictive algorithms. Neuroscience, perhaps, through defendant neuroimaging, may be able to increase the accuracy of these forecasts on its own or in combination with existing approaches [51].

Cognitive brain aging as a multidimensional geometric model. Each circle represents a set of variables that influence the multifaceted phenomena of aging.

Neuroscience could also aid in determining a person's current mental state. This could be highly useful in determining if a plaintiff is genuinely suffering from the crippling agony he claims. Every year, legal systems make millions of these judgments, frequently based on little more than the claimant's self-report. Neuroimaging findings that closely correlate with the presence or absence of subjective pain will almost certainly never be perfect. However, they may be far superior to our current tools. [52] Similarly, neuroscience may aid in determining whether a person knows something [53], has a certain emotional response to something, or is attempting to lie. Any of these methods of "mind-reading' could be incredibly beneficial in court, as well as in other situations. They will also create complicated constitutional concerns involving the Fourth [54] and Fifth [55] Amendments, at least in the United States.

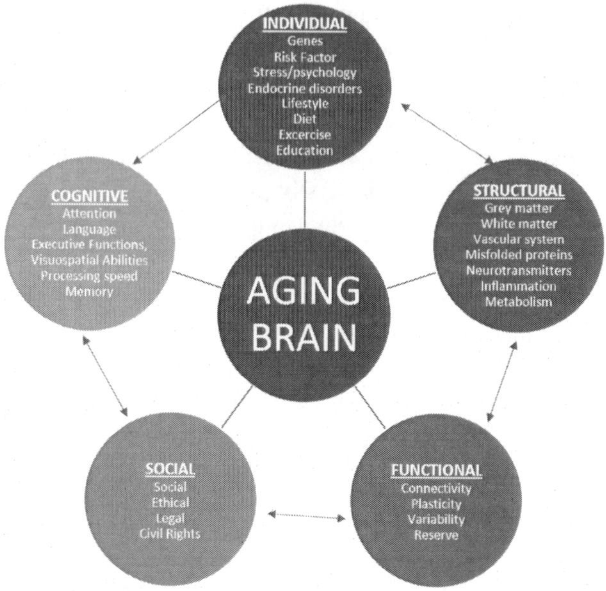

Figure 6. The parameters of brain aging.

When considering neuroscientific research in general, it is obvious that the greatest interest in and financing for neuroscience research is not motivated by enthusiasm for applications in prediction or detection. Instead, it is being propelled by hoped-for initiatives. We want medicines that can prevent, alleviate, or cure brain illness. Even though useful neuroscience interventions have been rare in the past, it is their optimism that drives this research. However, the essential issue for the law is that if we succeed in treating some types of disease, the level of understanding that this necessitates may also allow for the "treatment" of mental states that do not disorder. Shyness, sexual orientation, religiosity (or the lack thereof), and political opinions are among characteristics that some people might like to change in themselves or others. The legal and regulatory system will inevitably be involved in the cases where whether direct brain treatments are imposed by judges wanting to "rehabilitate" criminals, by parents seeking to "improve" their children, or by competent individuals seeking to "change their selves" [56].

Finally, neuroscience could open the path for new ways to improve mental abilities. The nonmedical use of Adderall or Ritalin for their (uncertain) cognitive boosting abilities has raised controversy. But what if medical research into disease treatments leads to the development of pharmaceuticals or devices that have been proven to improve health? How would we like such enhancements to be used in society and the judicial system in general? (Consider improving witnesses' memories or assisting students in passing the bar test.)

All such applicability of neuroscience, as well as others, will inevitably include the law. It will be asked to determine, interpret, and enforce the boundaries of behaviors made feasible by neuroscience in some cases. In other cases, neuroscience will have an impact on legal processes, ranging from the courtroom to the corporate lawyer's office to judge appointment difficulties. Law and neuroscience will become increasingly intertwined on issues that go far beyond responsibility, in one way or another.

Opportunities in Neurolaw

Neurolaw provides opportunities for psychiatry. Thus, "One of the most likely ways in which neuroscience may help the legal system" is the insanity defense [57]. In general, neuroscience could help with psychiatric evaluations of prisoners and defendants in three ways:

- Neuro-techniques can begin to help with the diagnostic process in psychiatry in the coming years. This could be extremely beneficial, especially since malingering is such a danger in forensic psychiatric evaluations. The defendant's comment should not be considered as granted. Neuroimaging could be used in the future to check or rule out a psychiatric analysis or psychopathological symptoms such as impulse control issues or grasp hallucinations [58],
- Neuroscience may aid in the prediction of future crimes. Predicting repetition in emotionally ill offenders is a fundamental goal of forensic psychiatry. Neuro-prediction could be a beneficial supplement for the current risk-assessment techniques, which have a very limited predictive value [59]. A greater risk assessment will result in the issue of many inmates and patients who are no longer dangerous and have better crime prevention,
- Neuroscience can be helpful not only to assess danger but also to recognize domains where involvements to minimize tendency in persons who are suffering from serious mental illness should be

focused. This would be tremendously beneficial not only to the patients but also to their families and society.

To summarise, intervention, prediction, and diagnosis are three areas where neuroscience could make a significant contribution to scientific psychoanalysis. Most likely, in the next years, there will be more intense arguments concerning the potential applications and consequences of neuroscience approaches in these fields.

Challenges in Neurolaw

Certain issues are faced by lawyers, society, and people under neurolaw.

There are two broad general categories under which challenges in neurolaw can be studied:

- Overenthusiasm,
- Over-criticism.

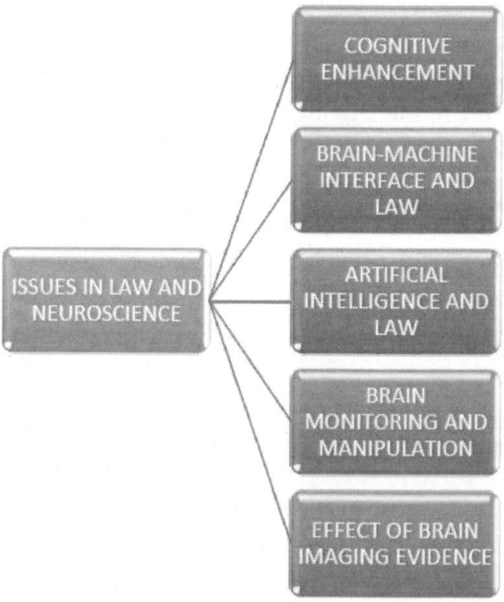

Figure 7. The issues in law and neuroscience.

Overenthusiasm

Because the use of neuroscience in the forensic psychiatric environment currently has major limits, overenthusiasm is a concern. One common criticism is that neuroscience tends to concentrate on groups, whereas the courtroom – at least in laws related to crimes – focuses on the individual, the offender [60]. At a group level, decreased hoary substance capacity in the prefrontal cortex can be linked to disruptive character disorder, but what does this signify for the individual defendant who has some hoary substance capacity reduction? In that case, a technique could be needed to help in the translation of conclusions at the group level to specific implications. Therefore, rather than enthusiasm, decades of biological psychiatry have led to a plea for modesty. Neurobiology has yet to play an important role in psychiatric diagnostic and treatment methods. Neuropsychiatric advances at a slower pace than expected and many of the findings are preliminary [61].

Ultimately, the neurolaw is often concerned with topics that neuroimaging or other research based on the brain cannot directly address. For example, men's rea (Latin word meaning "guilty mind", which refers to unlawful commitments) is a lawful idea that is not easily enclosed by neuroscientific or neuropsychiatric perceptions and methodology [62].

As a result, neuroscience findings must be taken with caution [63], not just because they are frequently introductory and worry the group level, but also because they may not directly discourse the lawful issue. Thus, necessitating the lawful issue requires additional interpretation and assumptions.

Overcriticism

Over-criticism is sometimes unproductive. We could be exposed to neuroscience's potential involvement in (forensic) psychiatry because it is such a massive and multi-layered endeavor. In forensic psychiatry, present valuations and decision-making are often distant from perfect. Diagnostic methods, therapy, and danger guess are all in desperate need of change [64].

We can't afford to ignore potentially beneficial neuroscience information and procedures. Psychiatrists are expected by their profession and society to use every tool at their fingertips to provide the best facilities conceivably. It could be imprudent and unreasonable to continue being uninvolved in neurolaw advancements [65], not just because the expansions may have much to give psychiatry, but also because psychiatrists have much to contribute to the neurolaw developments. The rationale for this is that some of them are concerned with problems that psychiatrists are well-versed in, like insanity determinations, interferences in emotionally ill offenders, and risk assessments. Over-criticism may have a catastrophic consequence, that psychiatrists will be excluded from neurolaw advancements.

Scope of Neurolaw in Future

Neuroscience can soon help in forensic psychiatrist analysis, forecast, and involvement. This opportunity could be regarded seriously, that is to say, it is not to be handled with either over-criticism or over-enthusiasm. Hence the goal of the neurolaw study is to strike a compromise between these two issues. If there is active participation by the psychiatrists in the developments, the chances of success will improve.

Conclusion

The intersection of neuroscience and law, also known as Neurolaw, is thought to provide practical transparency to the law and can assist the piece of legislation that regulates human behavior in holding justice and making it more rational.

The Neurolaw will assist lawyers in demonstrating to the judge the brain's functioning and its behavioral correlates which are beneficial for the case at hand. It will also assist lawyers in producing neuroscientific data to support an expert in presenting his opinion in the most scientifically sound manner possible to make justice more equitable.

However, there are other issues in the field of neurolaw that can be addressed through continuous research to understand, in short, how neuroscience affects jurisprudence. Even if the future of neurolaw is uncertain, it will aid in the proof of liability, expanding the scope of the law, improving a judge's knowledge in respect to a legal right, gaining a mature understanding of normative phenomena in terms of brain, mind and psychological insights, and revisiting various legal concepts and rules of liabilities and rights. It will also contribute to the expansion of the frontier of jurisprudence.

References

[1] Sayadmansour A. Neurotheology: The relationship between brain and religion. *Iran J Neurol.* 2014;13(1):52–5. [PMC free article] [PubMed] [Google Scholar].

[2] Bear MF, Connors BW, Paradiso MA. *Neuroscience.* Philadelphia, PA: Lippincott Williams & Wilkins; 2007. pp. 4–22. [Google Scholar].

[3] Wolf SM. Neurolaw: the big question. *Am J Bioeth.* 2008;8(1):21–2. [PubMed] [Google Scholar].

[4] Pardo MS, Patterson D. *Minds, Brains, and Law: The Conceptual Foundations of Law and Neuroscience.* Oxford, UK: Oxford University Press; 2013. pp. 23–4. [Google Scholar].

[5] Shafi N. Neuroscience and law: the evidentiary value of brain imaging. *Graduate Student Journal of Psychology.* 2009;11:27–39. [Google Scholar].

[6] Hart HL. *The Concept of Law.* Oxford, UK: Oxford University Press; 2012. [Google Scholar].

[7] Cohler AM, Miller BC, Stone HS. *Montesquieu: The Spirit of the Laws.* Cambridge, UK: Cambridge University Press; 1989. [Google Scholar].

[8] Bigler ED. Neuropsychological assessment, neuroimaging, and clinical neuropsychology: a synthesis. *Arch Clin Neuropsychol.* 1991;6(3):113–32. [PubMed] [Google Scholar].

[9] Baskin JH, Edersheim JG, Price BH. Is a picture worth a thousand words? Neuroimaging in the courtroom. *Am J Law Med.* 2007;33(2-3):239–69. [PubMed] [Google Scholar].

[10] Tovino SA. Functional neuroimaging and the law: trends and directions for future scholarship. *Am J Bioeth.* 2007;7(9):44–56. [PubMed] [Google Scholar].

[11] Takahashi T. Molecular neuroeconomics of crime and punishment: implications for neurolaw. *Neuro Endocrinol Lett.* 2012;33(7):667–73. [PubMed] [Google Scholar].

[12] Poldrack RA. Mapping mental function to brain structure: How can cognitive neuroimaging succeed? *Perspect Psychol Sci.* 2010;5(5):753–61. [PMC free article] [PubMed] [Google Scholar].

[13] Mohr PN, Nagel IE. Variability in brain activity as an individual difference measure in neuroscience? *J Neurosci.* 2010;30(23):7755–7. [PMC free article] [PubMed] [Google Scholar].

[14] Meynen G. Neurolaw: neuroscience, ethics, and law. Review essay. *Ethical Theory Moral Pract.* 2014;17:819–29. [Google Scholar].

[15] Greely HT. Mind reading, neuroscience, and the law. In: *A Primer on Criminal Law and Neuroscience. A contribution to the law and neuroscience project, supported by the MacArthur Foundation.* New York: Oxford University Press; 2013. [Google Scholar].

[16] Pardo MS, Patterson D. Minds, brains, and law. *The Conceptual Foundations of Law and Neuroscience.* New York: Oxford University Press; 2013. [Google Scholar].

[17] Fuss J, Auer MK, Biedermann SV, et al. Deep brain stimulation to reduce sexual drive. *J Psychiatry Neurosci.* 2015;40:429–31. [PMC free article] [PubMed] [Google Scholar].

[18] Gasson MN, Koops BJ. Attacking human implants: a new generation of cybercrime. *Law, Innovation, and Technology*. 2013;5:248–77. [Google Scholar].
[19] Jones EG, Mendell LM. Assessing the decade of the brain. *Science*. 1999;284(5415):739. [PubMed] [Google Scholar].
[20] Taylor JS, Harp JA, Elliott T. Neuropsychologists and neurolawyers. *Neuropsychology*. 1991;5(4):293–305. [Google Scholar].
[21] Taylor JS. Neurolaw: towards a new medical jurisprudence. *Brain Inj.* 1995;9(7):745–51. [PubMed] [Google Scholar].
[22] MacArthur Foundation. The future of law and neuroscience [Online] [cited 2013 Apr 27]. Available from: URL: http://www.lawneuro.org/aba/index.php.
[23] Vincent NA. *Neuroscience and Legal Responsibility*. Oxford, UK: Oxford University Press; 2013. [Google Scholar].
[24] Spranger TM. *International Neurolaw: A Comparative Analysis*. Berlin, Germany: Springer Science & Business Media; 2012. [Google Scholar].
[25] Pennsylvania Trial Lawyers Association. *Neurolaw for Trial Lawyers: Closed Head Injuries, Neuromuscular Diseases, Reflex Sympathetic Dystrophy & Beyond*. Philadelphia, PA: Pennsylvania Trial Lawyers Association; 1994. [Google Scholar].
[26] Freeman M. *Law and Neuroscience: Current Legal Issues*. Oxford, UK: Oxford University Press; 2011. [Google Scholar].
[27] Uttal WR. *Neuroscience in the Courtroom: What Every Lawyer Should Know About the Mind and the Brain*. Tucson, AZ: Lawyers and Judges Publishing Company; 2009. [Google Scholar].
[28] Morse SJ, Roskies AL. *A Primer on Criminal Law and Neuroscience: A Contribution of the Law and Neuroscience Project, Supported by the MacArthur Foundation*. Oxford, UK: Oxford University Press; 2013. [Google Scholar].
[29] Pardo MS, Patterson D. *Minds, Brains, and Law: The Conceptual Foundations of Law and Neuroscience*. Oxford, UK: Oxford University Press; 2013. pp. 23–4. [Google Scholar].
[30] Taylor JS. *Neurolaw: Brain and Spinal Cord Injuries*. New York, NY: Clark Boardman Callaghan; 1997. [Google Scholar].
[31] Freeman MD, Goodenough OR. *Law, Mind, and Brain*. Farnham, UK: Ashgate Publishing, Ltd; 2009. [Google Scholar].
[32] Taylor JS, Harp JA, Elliott T. *Materials on Neurolaw*. London, UK: Taylor & Harp; 1991. [Google Scholar].
[33] Goodenough OR, Zeki S. *Law, and the Brain*. Oxford, UK: Oxford University Press; 2006. [Google Scholar].
[34] Glicksohn J. *The Neurobiology of Criminal Behavior*. Berlin, Germany: Springer Science & Business Media; 2002. [Google Scholar].
[35] Church, D. (2011). Neuroscience in the courtroom: an international concern. *Wm. Mary L. Rev*. 53, 1825–1854.
[36] Gaudet, L. M. (2011). Brain fingerprinting, scientific evidence, and "daubert": a cautionary lesson from India. *Jurimetrics*, 51(3), 293–318.
[37] Bles, M., and Haynes, J. (2008). Detecting concealed information using brain-imaging technology. *Neurocase* 14, 82–92. DOI: 10.1080/13554790801992784.

[38] Brown, T., and Murphy, E. (2010). Through a scanner darkly: functional neuroimaging as evidence of a criminal defendant's past mental states. *Stanf. Law Rev.* 62, 1119–1208.

[39] Parmar, V., & Mukundan, C.R. (2017). Brain Electrical Oscillation Signature Profiling (BEOS). *International Journal of Computers in Clinical Practice,* 2(1), 1–24.

[40] Bernstein, D., and Jackson, J. (2004). The Daubert trilogy in the states. *Jurimetrics* 44, 351–366.

[41] Alexander, A. (2007). Functional magnetic resonance imaging lie detection: is a brainstorm headed for the gatekeeper? *Houst. J. Health L. Policy* 7, 1–56.

[42] Davatzikos, C., Ruparel, K., Fan, Y., Shen, D. G., Acharyya, M., Loughead, J. W., et al. (2005). Classifying spatial patterns of brain activity with machine learning methods: application to lie detection. *NeuroImage* 28, 663–668. doi: 10.1016/j.neuroimage.2005.08.009.

[43] Ghiridharadas, A. (2008). India's novel use of brain scans in court is debated. *New York Times*, Sept 14, 14:A10.

[44] Henry T. Greely and Nita A. Farahany (2019). Neuroscience and the Criminal Justice System. *Annual Review of Criminology* 2:1, 451-471.

[45] Aono, D., Yaffe, G., & Kober, H. (2019). Neuroscientific evidence in the courtroom: a review. *Cognitive Research: Principles and Implications*, 4(1), 40.

[46] Jones OD, Marois R, Farah MJ, Greely HT. (2013). Law and neuroscience. *The Journal of Neuroscience* 33(45):17624–30. [PMC free article] [PubMed] [Google Scholar].

[47] Jones OD. Seven ways neuroscience aids law [Online] [cited 2013]. Available from: http://www.casinapioiv.va/content/dam/accademia/pdf/sv121/sv121-jones.pdf.

[48] Sahakian B, Morein-Zamir S. Professor's little helper. (200..) *Nature.* 450(7173): 1157–9. [PubMed] [Google Scholar].

[49] MacArthur Foundation. The future of law and neuroscience [Online] [cited 2013 Apr 27]. Available from: http://www.lawneuro.org/aba/index.php.

[50] Greely HT (2009). Law and the revolution in neuroscience: an early look at the field. *Akron L Rev* 42:687–715. [Google Scholar].

[51] Aharoni E, Vincent GM, Harenski CL, Calhoun VD, Sinnott-Armstrong W, Gazzaniga MS, Kiehl KA (2012). Neuroprediction of future rearrest. *Proc Natl Acad Sci USA* 110:6223–6228, doi:10.1073/pnas.1219302110, pmid:23536303. [CrossRef] [PubMed] [Google Scholar].

[52] Kolber AJ (2007). Pain detection and the privacy of subjective experience. *Am J L Med* 33:433–456. [Google Scholar].

[53] Meixner JB, Rosenfeld JP (2011) A mock terrorism application of the P300-based concealed information test. *Psychophysiology* 48:149–154, doi:10.1111/j.1469-8986.2010.01050.x. [CrossRef] [Google Scholar].

[54] Farahany N (2012). Searching secrets. *Penn L Rev* 160:1239–1308. [Google Scholar].

[55] Farahany N (2012). Incriminating thoughts. *Stanford L Rev* 64:351–408. [Google Scholar].

[56] Greely HT (2008). Neuroscience and criminal justice: not responsibility but treatment. *Univ Kans L Rev* 56:1103–1138. [Google Scholar].

[57] Meynen G. (2013). A neurolaw perspective on psychiatric assessments of criminal responsibility: decision-making, mental disorder, and the brain. *Int J Law Psychiatry* 36:93–9. [PubMed] [Google Scholar].

[58] Meynen G. (2014) Neurolaw: de relevantie voor de forensische psychiatrie. *Tijdschr Psychiatr* 56:597–604. [PubMed] [Google Scholar].

[59] Nadelhoffer T, Bibas S, Grafton S, et al. (2012). Neuroprediction, violence, and the law: setting the stage. *Neuroethics* 5:67–99. [PMC free article] [PubMed] [Google Scholar].

[60] Buckholtz JW, Faigman DL. (2014). Promises, promises for neuroscience and law. *Curr Biol* 24:R861–7. [PubMed] [Google Scholar].

[61] Rose NS, Abi-Rached JM. *Neuro: The New Brain Sciences and the Management of the Mind.* Princeton: Princeton University Press; 2013. [Google Scholar].

[62] Meynen G. Neuroethics of criminal responsibility: mental disorders influencing behavior. In: *The Routledge International Handbook of Biosocial Criminology.* Abingdon: Routledge; 2015. pp. 544–557. [Google Scholar].

[63] Morse SJ, Roskies AL. *A Primer on Criminal Law and Neuroscience: A Contribution of the Law and Neuroscience Project, Supported by the MacArthur Foundation.* New York: Oxford University Press; 2013. [Google Scholar].

[64] Meynen G. A neurolaw perspective on psychiatric assessments of criminal responsibility: decision-making, mental disorder, and the brain. *Int J Law Psychiatry.* 2013;36:93–9. [PubMed] [Google Scholar].

[65] Silva JA. The relevance of neuroscience to forensic psychiatry. *J Am Acad Psychiatry Law.* 2007;35:6–9. [PubMed] [Google Scholar].

Editors' Contact Information

Dr. Prachi Srivastava
Assistant Professor, Amity Institute of Biotechnology,
Amity University, Lucknow, Uttar Pradesh, India
Email: psrivastava@amity.edu.

Dr. Neha Srivastava
Associate Scientist, Computational Biology (Pharma Analytics)
Excelra Knowledge Solution Pvt Ltd.
NSL Arena, Uppal, Hyderabad, India
Email: ns011982@gmail.com.

Prekshi Garg
Research Scholar, Amity Institute of Biotechnology,
Amity University, Lucknow, Uttar Pradesh, India
Email: prekshigarg23@gmail.com.

Index

O

P

Q

R

S

T

U

V

W

X